GETTING A COLONOSCOPY

Your Guide to Preparation, a Pain-Free
Procedure, and Peace of Mind

BY ETHAN D. ANDERSON

WWW.BORNINCREDIBLE.COM

Table of Contents

Introduction

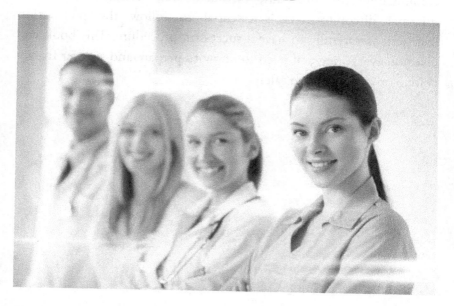

"So You're Getting A Colonoscopy: Everything You Need To Know To Prepare and Recover from a Colonoscopy Quickly and Safely" is a comprehensive guide that provides you with detailed information on the colonoscopy procedure, including how to prepare for the procedure, what to expect during the procedure, and how to recover from it.

A colonoscopy is a procedure where a doctor inserts a long, flexible tube with a camera into the rectum and large intestine to check for problems. It is also used to remove polyps, which are abnormal growths that could become cancerous.

You may feel a bit nervous if you have been scheduled for a colonoscopy. This procedure is usually well tolerated and causes minimal discomfort. It is essential to follow the preparation instructions carefully to have a successful procedure. This book will give you everything you need to know to prepare and recover from a colonoscopy quickly and safely.

What is a colonoscopy?

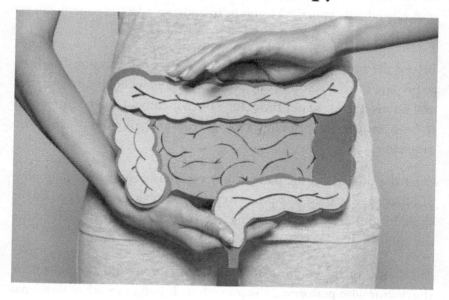

A colonoscopy is a medical procedure that allows a doctor to examine the inside of the colon, also known as the large intestine. This procedure is typically used to detect and diagnose colon cancer, as well as other conditions such as polyps, inflammatory bowel disease, and diverticulitis.

During the procedure, a long, flexible tube called a colonoscope is inserted into the rectum and gradually advanced through the colon. The colonoscope has a small camera and light on the end, which allows the doctor to view the inside of the colon on a monitor. The doctor may also use small instruments through the scope to remove polyps or take biopsies.

The procedure is performed while the patient is under sedation, which means they are awake but relaxed and comfortable. The procedure typically takes between 30 minutes to an hour, and the patient can go home the same day.

Before the procedure, the patient will be given instructions on how to prepare for the colonoscopy, which typically includes a special diet and laxatives to clean out the colon. The patient will also be instructed to stop eating and drinking a certain number of hours before the procedure.

After the procedure, the patient may experience some mild cramping or bloating, but these symptoms typically resolve quickly. The patient should avoid driving or operating heavy machinery for the rest of the day and should have someone to accompany them home.

The results of the colonoscopy will be discussed with the patient by the doctor who performed the procedure. If polyps or other abnormal growths are found, they will be removed during the procedure or biopsied for further testing. If cancer is found, the patient will be referred to a specialist for further treatment.

Colonoscopy is a safe and effective procedure, but as with any medical procedure, there are some risks. These can include bleeding, infection, and perforation of the colon. The risk of complications is generally low, but it is important to discuss any concerns with the doctor before the procedure.

Overall, a colonoscopy is an important tool in the detection and diagnosis of colon cancer and other conditions affecting the colon. It is recommended for individuals over the age of 50 or for those with a family history of colon cancer, and it is usually performed every 10 years. It can be uncomfortable, but it is a minor inconvenience for the peace of mind and early detection it can bring.

Understanding Colonoscopy

Colonoscopy is a medical procedure that involves the examination of the colon or large intestine using a flexible, lighted tube known as a colonoscope. The purpose of this procedure is to screen for colorectal cancer, identify and remove any polyps, and investigate the cause of various gastrointestinal symptoms.

Despite its importance in diagnosing and preventing colorectal cancer, many people are still hesitant about getting a colonoscopy due to the fear of discomfort, embarrassment, and inconvenience associated with the procedure. In this article, we will provide a detailed understanding of colonoscopy to help you overcome these fears and make informed decisions about your health.

Preparation for Colonoscopy

Before the colonoscopy procedure, you will need to follow specific instructions to prepare your bowel for the examination. This process involves cleaning your colon thoroughly to remove any fecal matter or debris that may interfere with the visibility of the colonoscope.

Your doctor will provide you with a set of instructions on what to eat and drink in the days leading up to the procedure. This typically includes a low-fiber diet and a clear liquid diet for at least 24 hours before the colonoscopy. You will also need to take laxatives or other bowel-cleansing agents to help clear your colon.

The colonoscopy procedure is typically performed under sedation, which means that you will be asleep or in a drowsy state during the examination. However, it is essential to have someone drive you home after the procedure as the sedative effects can last for several hours.

During the Colonoscopy

During the colonoscopy procedure, you will lie on your side with your knees bent towards your chest. Your doctor will insert the colonoscope through your anus and slowly advance it into your colon while inflating your colon with air to allow for a better view.

The colonoscope has a tiny camera attached to its tip that transmits images of your colon to a monitor in the exam room. This allows your doctor to examine the inside of your colon for any abnormal growths, polyps, inflammation, or other issues.

If your doctor identifies any polyps during the examination, they may remove them using specialized tools inserted through the colonoscope. The removed polyps are then sent to a laboratory for further analysis to determine if they are cancerous or precancerous.

The entire colonoscopy procedure usually takes between 30 minutes to an hour, depending on the complexity of your colon and any issues that your doctor may find.

After the Colonoscopy

After the colonoscopy, you may experience some mild cramping, bloating, or gas due to the air that was introduced into your colon during the procedure. This is typically temporary and should subside within a few hours.

It is essential to follow your doctor's post-procedure instructions carefully to ensure a smooth recovery. This may include avoiding solid foods for a few hours and gradually resuming your regular diet over the next few days.

Your doctor will also provide you with instructions on how to care for your anus and rectum after the procedure. This typically includes avoiding strenuous activity, taking a warm bath, and using a soothing ointment to reduce any discomfort or irritation.

Why is Colonoscopy Important?

Colonoscopy is an essential screening tool for the early detection and prevention of colorectal cancer, which is the third most common cancer in the United States. According to the American Cancer Society, colorectal cancer is expected to cause over 52,000 deaths in the United States in 2021 alone.

Screening for colorectal cancer using colonoscopy is recommended for people aged 50 and above, or earlier if you have a family history of colorectal cancer, inflammatory bowel disease, or other risk factors. Regular colonoscopy screenings can help detect and remove precancerous polyps before the mutate into something more dangerous.

Definition and Purpose

Colonoscopy is a medical procedure that allows doctors to examine the colon or large intestine using a flexible, lighted tube known as a colonoscope. The purpose of this procedure is to screen for colorectal cancer, identify and remove any polyps, and investigate the cause of various gastrointestinal symptoms.

The colon is an essential part of the digestive system that absorbs water and nutrients from the food we eat. However, the colon can also be the site of various diseases, including colorectal cancer, inflammatory bowel disease, diverticulitis, and other conditions that can cause abdominal pain, bloating, diarrhea, constipation, and other symptoms.

Colonoscopy is an effective tool for detecting and preventing these diseases, and it is recommended for people aged 50 and above, or earlier if you have a family history of colorectal cancer, inflammatory bowel disease, or other risk factors.

How Does Colonoscopy Work?

Colonoscopy involves the use of a colonoscope, which is a long, flexible tube with a tiny camera and light attached to its tip. The colonoscope is inserted through the anus and advanced slowly into the colon while inflating it with air to allow for a better view.

The camera on the colonoscope transmits images of the inside of the colon to a monitor in the exam room, allowing the doctor to examine the lining of the colon for any abnormalities, including polyps, inflammation, or other issues.

If the doctor finds any polyps during the examination, they may remove them using specialized tools inserted through the colonoscope. The removed polyps are then sent to a laboratory for further analysis to determine if they are cancerous or precancerous.

Why is Colonoscopy Important?

Colonoscopy is an essential screening tool for the early detection and prevention of colorectal cancer, which is the third most common cancer in the United States. According to the American Cancer Society, colorectal cancer is expected to cause over 52,000 deaths in the United States in 2021 alone.

Screening for colorectal cancer using colonoscopy is recommended for people aged 50 and above, or earlier if you have a family history of colorectal cancer, inflammatory bowel disease, or other risk factors. Regular colonoscopy screenings can help detect and remove precancerous polyps before they develop into cancer, reducing the risk of developing colorectal cancer.

In addition to screening for colorectal cancer, colonoscopy can also be used to investigate the cause of various gastrointestinal symptoms, such as abdominal pain, diarrhea, constipation, and rectal bleeding. Colonoscopy can help diagnose conditions such as inflammatory bowel disease, diverticulitis, and other gastrointestinal conditions.

Preparing for Colonoscopy

Preparing for a colonoscopy is essential to ensure that the procedure is successful and that the doctor can get a clear view of the inside of the colon. The preparation process involves cleaning the colon to remove any fecal matter or debris that may interfere with the visibility of the colonoscope.

Your doctor will provide you with specific instructions on what to eat and drink in the days leading up to the procedure. This typically includes a low-fiber diet and a clear liquid diet for at least 24 hours before the colonoscopy. You will also need to take laxatives or other bowel-cleansing agents to help clear your colon.

It is essential to follow these instructions carefully to ensure that the colonoscopy is successful and that the doctor can get a clear view of the inside of the colon.

During Colonoscopy

During the colonoscopy procedure, you will lie on your side with your knees bent towards your chest. The doctor will insert the colonoscope through your anus and slowly advance it into your colon while inflating your colon with air to allow for a better view.

Colonoscopy vs

When it comes to screening for colorectal cancer, there are several options available, including colonoscopy, stool-based tests, and virtual colonoscopy. Each of these tests has its advantages and disadvantages, and the choice of which one to undergo depends on several factors, including personal preferences, medical history, and the risk of developing colorectal cancer.

In this article, we will compare colonoscopy, the gold standard in colorectal cancer screening, with other screening options to help you make an informed decision about which screening test is best for you.

Colonoscopy

Colonoscopy is a medical procedure that involves the examination of the colon or large intestine using a flexible, lighted tube known as a colonoscope. The purpose of this procedure is to screen for colorectal cancer, identify and remove any polyps, and investigate the cause of various gastrointestinal symptoms.

Colonoscopy is considered the gold standard in colorectal cancer screening as it provides a direct visualization of the colon and allows for the removal of any precancerous polyps during the procedure. The procedure is typically performed under sedation, which means that you will be asleep or in a drowsy state during the examination.

Colonoscopy is recommended for people aged 50 and above, or earlier if you have a family history of colorectal cancer, inflammatory bowel disease, or other risk factors. The procedure is typically performed every 10 years, although the frequency may be higher for those at higher risk of developing colorectal cancer.

Stool-based Tests

Stool-based tests are non-invasive tests that detect the presence of blood or abnormal cells in the stool. These tests are designed to identify the presence of precancerous polyps or early-stage colorectal cancer.

There are several types of stool-based tests available, including fecal immunochemical test (FIT), fecal occult blood test (FOBT), and stool DNA test.

FIT and FOBT are designed to detect blood in the stool, which can be an early sign of colorectal cancer. These tests involve collecting a stool sample at home and sending it to a laboratory for analysis. If blood is detected in the stool, a follow-up colonoscopy is usually recommended to confirm the diagnosis and identify the source of the bleeding.

Stool DNA test, on the other hand, detects the presence of abnormal cells in the stool, which can be an early sign of colorectal cancer. This test involves collecting a stool sample at home and sending it to a laboratory for analysis. If abnormal cells are detected in the stool, a follow-up colonoscopy is usually recommended to confirm the diagnosis and identify the location of the abnormal cells.

Stool-based tests are typically recommended for people who are unable or unwilling to undergo colonoscopy. These tests are also recommended for people who are at average risk of developing colorectal cancer.

Virtual Colonoscopy

Virtual colonoscopy, also known as computed tomography (CT) colonography, is a non-invasive procedure that uses X-rays to create detailed images of the colon. The images are then used to create a 3D model of the colon, which allows doctors to examine the colon for any abnormalities.

Virtual colonoscopy is typically performed every five years, although the frequency may be higher for those at higher risk of developing colorectal cancer.

Virtual colonoscopy is considered less invasive than colonoscopy as it does not require the insertion of a colonoscope into the rectum. However, like colonoscopy, virtual colonoscopy requires bowel preparation, which involves cleaning the colon to remove any fecal matter or debris that may interfere with the visibility of the colon.

A virtual colonoscopy is recommended for people who are unable or unwilling to undergo colonoscopy or who are at average risk of developing colorectal cancer.

Expert Advice

Expert Advice: What You Need to Know Before Getting a Colonoscopy

Colonoscopy is a commonly performed medical procedure used to detect abnormalities in the large intestine or colon, including polyps and colorectal cancer. While it can be a life-saving procedure, many people are nervous or apprehensive about getting a colonoscopy. To help ease these concerns, we've compiled some expert advice on what you need to know before getting a colonoscopy.

Why is colonoscopy important?

Colonoscopy is an important screening tool for colorectal cancer, which is the second leading cause of cancer-related deaths in the United States. Colorectal cancer often develops from precancerous polyps in the colon or rectum, which can be removed during a colonoscopy before they have a chance to turn into cancer.

"Colonoscopy is the gold standard for colon cancer screening," says Dr. David Johnson, a gastroenterologist and former president of the American College of Gastroenterology. "It allows us to detect and remove polyps that could turn into cancer, and it's the only test that can do that."

Who should get a colonoscopy?

The American Cancer Society recommends that people at average risk of colorectal cancer start regular screening at age 45. However, some people may need to start screening earlier if they have certain risk factors, such as a family history of colorectal cancer or a personal history of inflammatory bowel disease.

"You should talk to your doctor about when to start screening and how often to get screened," says Dr. Johnson. "Your doctor will take into account your personal and family medical history, as well as other factors that may affect your risk of colorectal cancer."

What should I expect during the colonoscopy?

During a colonoscopy, a long, flexible tube with a tiny camera at the end (called a colonoscope) is inserted into the rectum and advanced through the colon. This allows the doctor to view the inside of the colon and rectum and look for any abnormalities. If any polyps or other abnormalities are found, they can be removed during the procedure.

"You will be given a sedative to help you relax and a pain medication to reduce discomfort," says Dr. Johnson. "The procedure itself usually takes about 30-60 minutes, and most people are able to go home a few hours afterward."

What are the potential risks of colonoscopy?

Like any medical procedure, colonoscopy carries some risks. The most serious risk is perforation (a tear or hole) in the colon, which can require surgery to repair. Other potential risks include bleeding, infection, and reaction to sedation.

"Although the risk of complications is small, it's important to discuss the potential risks and benefits of colonoscopy with your doctor before the procedure," says Dr. Johnson. "Your doctor will also give you instructions on how to prepare for the procedure, such as fasting and taking laxatives to clear out the colon."

Are there any alternatives to colonoscopy?

While colonoscopy is the gold standard for colorectal cancer screening, there are other options available. These include:

2. Fecal immunochemical test (FIT): This test detects blood in the stool, which can be a sign of colorectal cancer. It is done at home and mailed to a lab for analysis.

3. Stool DNA test: This test looks for DNA changes in cells shed by polyps or cancer in the stool. It is also done at home and mailed to a lab for analysis.

4. CT colonography: This test uses X-rays and computer technology to create detailed images of the colon. It is less invasive than colonoscopy but still requires bowel preparation and may not be covered by insurance.

"Talk to your doctor about which screening test is right for for your situation.

Common Concerns

Colonoscopy is an important diagnostic tool used for screening, diagnosing, and treating various conditions of the colon and rectum. However, despite its proven effectiveness, many people have concerns and fears regarding the procedure. In this article, we will address some of the common concerns and questions about colonoscopy.

Is colonoscopy painful?

One of the most common concerns about colonoscopy is the fear of pain. However, the procedure is generally not painful. Before the procedure, patients are usually given sedatives or anesthesia to help them relax and reduce discomfort. During the procedure, patients may feel some pressure or discomfort, but this is typically mild and transient.

How long does colonoscopy take?

The length of the procedure varies depending on the individual case, but generally, it takes around 30 minutes to an hour. However, additional time may be needed if polyps or other abnormalities are detected and removed.

How should I prepare for colonoscopy?

Preparation for colonoscopy usually involves a special diet and cleansing of the colon. Patients are instructed to follow a low-fiber diet for several days before the procedure and to consume a special solution to clean the colon. It is important to follow the instructions provided by the doctor or medical staff to ensure a successful procedure.

Can I eat after colonoscopy?

After the procedure, patients are usually advised to avoid solid foods until the effects of the sedative or anesthesia wear off. However, they may drink clear liquids and gradually resume a normal diet as tolerated.

How often should I have a colonoscopy?

The frequency of colonoscopy depends on individual risk factors and previous findings. For average-risk individuals, it is recommended to have a colonoscopy every 10 years starting at age 50. However, for individuals with a family history of colon cancer or other risk factors, more frequent screenings may be recommended.

What are the risks of colonoscopy?

While colonoscopy is generally safe, there are some potential risks. These include bleeding, infection, perforation, and adverse reactions to sedatives or anesthesia. However, these risks are rare and can usually be managed with proper care and monitoring.

Can I drive after colonoscopy?

Due to the effects of the sedative or anesthesia, patients are usually advised not to drive or operate machinery for at least 24 hours after the procedure. It is important to arrange for transportation to and from the medical facility and to have someone stay with you during the recovery period.

What should I do if I have concerns about colonoscopy?

If you have concerns or questions about colonoscopy, it is important to discuss them with your doctor or medical provider. They can provide you with information and guidance to help you feel more comfortable and confident about the procedure.

Misconceptions about Colonoscopy

Colonoscopy is a medical procedure that involves inserting a flexible tube with a camera on the end into the colon to examine it for any abnormalities. Despite its effectiveness in detecting and preventing colorectal cancer, many people are reluctant to undergo the procedure due to various misconceptions. Below we will address some of the most common misconceptions about colonoscopy and provide factual information to help alleviate any concerns.

1. Misconception #1: Colonoscopy is a painful and uncomfortable procedure.

The truth is, most patients who undergo colonoscopy experience very little discomfort. The procedure is typically performed under sedation, which means you will be asleep or in a deep state of relaxation during the procedure. Additionally, the use of lubricants and gentle techniques by experienced medical professionals can help minimize any discomfort or pain. After the procedure, you may experience some cramping or bloating, but these symptoms usually subside within a few hours.

2. Misconception #2: Colonoscopy is embarrassing.

It is natural to feel a bit uncomfortable about the idea of having a medical professional examine your colon, but it is important to remember that the procedure is performed in a private room and medical professionals are trained to be respectful and considerate. Additionally, the benefits of having a colonoscopy far outweigh any potential embarrassment or discomfort.

3. Misconception #3: Colonoscopy is only necessary for people with a family history of colorectal cancer.

While having a family history of colorectal cancer is certainly a risk factor, anyone can develop colorectal cancer regardless of family history. The American Cancer Society recommends that everyone begin regular screening for colorectal cancer starting at age 45, or earlier if you have a family history or other risk factors. Regular screening is crucial because it can detect colorectal cancer in its early stages when it is more easily treated.

4. Misconception #4: Colonoscopy is unnecessary if I have no symptoms.

Many people mistakenly believe that if they have no symptoms, they do not need to undergo colonoscopy. However, colorectal cancer often has no symptoms in its early stages. By the time symptoms develop, the cancer may have already advanced, making it more difficult to treat. Regular screening can help detect colorectal cancer before it has a chance to progress, improving the chances of successful treatment.

5. Misconception #5: I do not need to prepare for colonoscopy.

Preparing for colonoscopy is an important part of the procedure. The colon must be completely empty so that the camera can get a clear view of the colon lining. Your healthcare provider will provide instructions on how to prepare for the procedure, which usually involves following a special diet and taking laxatives to help clear out your colon.

6. Misconception #6: Colonoscopy is not covered by insurance.

In fact, most health insurance plans cover the cost of colonoscopy as a preventive screening test. The Affordable Care Act requires most health plans to cover the cost of preventive screenings, including colonoscopy, without charging a copayment or coinsurance. If you are concerned about the cost of the procedure, it is best to speak with your insurance provider to confirm your coverage.

7. Misconception #7: Colonoscopy is a one-time procedure.

While colonoscopy is an effective tool for detecting and preventing colorectal cancer, it is not a one-time procedure. The frequency of screening depends on various factors, such as age, family history, and personal health history. Your healthcare provider can help determine the appropriate screening interval for you.

Does it hurt to have a colonoscopy?

The most common question people have before having a colonoscopy is whether or not it will hurt. The answer is that it can cause some discomfort, but most people do not find the procedure to be painful.

Before the procedure, a patient will typically be given a sedative to help them relax and a medication called a laxative to clean out the colon. The sedative will make the patient feel drowsy and less aware of what is happening during the procedure, but they will still be able to respond to the doctor's instructions. The laxative will cause diarrhea, which can be uncomfortable, but it is important for the procedure to be as thorough as possible.

During the procedure, the patient will lie on their side on an examination table and the doctor will insert the colonoscope into the rectum. The tube is gently moved through the large intestine, while the doctor watches the images on a screen to look for any abnormalities. Air is also pumped into the colon to help the doctor see better. This can cause some cramping and bloating, but the sedative should help to reduce any discomfort. The entire procedure usually takes around 30 minutes to an hour.

After the procedure, the patient may feel some discomfort and bloating due to the air that was pumped into the colon, but this should pass quickly. They may also feel a bit groggy from the sedative, but this should wear off within a couple of hours. The patient may also experience some rectal bleeding or mild cramps for a day or two after the procedure but this is normal.

Overall, a colonoscopy is considered a safe and effective procedure for detecting colon cancer and other conditions. It can cause some discomfort, but most people do not find it to be painful. If you are scheduled for a colonoscopy, it is important to discuss any concerns you may have with your doctor and to follow their instructions for preparation and aftercare to ensure the best possible outcome.

Why might someone need a colonoscopy?

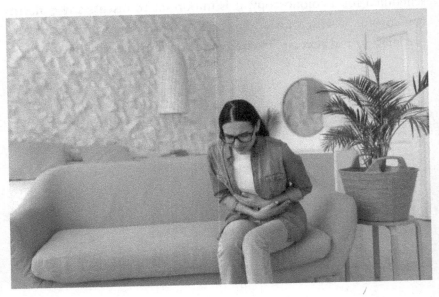

A colonoscopy is a medical procedure in which a doctor uses a thin, flexible tube with a camera at the end, called a colonoscope, to examine the inside of the colon and rectum. The procedure is used to detect and diagnose a variety of conditions and diseases affecting the large intestine, including colon cancer, inflammatory bowel disease (IBD), and polyps (small growths on the lining of the colon or rectum).

One of the primary reasons someone may need a colonoscopy is to screen for colon cancer. Colon cancer is the third most common cancer in men and women in the United States, and the second leading cause of cancer deaths. Screening for colon cancer can detect precancerous polyps, which can be removed before they turn into cancer, or early-stage cancer, which is more likely to be successfully treated. The American Cancer Society recommends that people at average risk of colon cancer begin screening at age 45, and that people at increased risk, such as those with a family history of colon cancer or a personal history of precancerous polyps, begin screening earlier.

Another reason someone may need a colonoscopy is to investigate symptoms that may be indicative of a problem with the large intestine. These symptoms can include rectal bleeding, abdominal pain, changes in bowel habits, and unexplained weight loss. A colonoscopy allows the doctor to examine the inside of the colon and rectum to look for the cause of these symptoms and make a diagnosis.

Inflammatory bowel disease (IBD), which includes Crohn's disease and ulcerative colitis, is another condition that may be diagnosed and monitored with a colonoscopy. These conditions cause inflammation and ulceration of the lining of the colon and rectum, and can lead to symptoms such as abdominal pain, diarrhea, and bleeding. A colonoscopy can help the doctor evaluate the extent and severity of the inflammation and make a diagnosis.

Other reasons someone may need a colonoscopy include the following:

Follow-up after treatment for colon cancer or precancerous polyps: After treatment, a colonoscopy may be performed to ensure that all of the abnormal tissue has been removed, and to monitor for any recurrence.

Evaluation of anemia: Anemia is a condition in which there is a decrease in the number of red blood cells or hemoglobin in the blood. Anemia can be caused by bleeding from the colon or rectum, and a colonoscopy can be used to find the source of the bleeding.

Evaluation of chronic diarrhea: A colonoscopy can be used to evaluate the cause of chronic diarrhea, which can be a symptom of many conditions, including IBD, celiac disease, and infections.

Evaluation of unexplained weight loss: Unexplained weight loss can be caused by many conditions, including cancer. A colonoscopy can be used to evaluate the cause of weight loss and rule out cancer as a possible cause.

Overall, a colonoscopy is a useful procedure that allows doctors to detect and diagnose a variety of conditions and diseases affecting the large intestine. It is particularly important for screening for colon cancer, which can be successfully treated if caught early. The procedure is also used to investigate symptoms and monitor conditions such as IBD. It's important to follow the guidelines of your doctor and health organization for the recommended schedule of colonoscopy.

Reasons to have a Colonoscopy

Colonoscopy is a medical procedure that allows doctors to examine the colon or large intestine for any abnormalities, including polyps, inflammation, or other issues. The procedure is an essential tool for the early detection and prevention of colorectal cancer, the third most common cancer in the United States. Here are some of the top reasons to consider having a colonoscopy:

1. Screen for Colorectal Cancer: Colonoscopy is the gold standard in colorectal cancer screening, allowing doctors to detect and remove precancerous polyps before they develop into cancer.

2. Family History of Colorectal Cancer: If you have a family history of colorectal cancer, you may be at a higher risk of developing the disease. Colonoscopy is recommended for people with a family history of colorectal cancer, and screening may begin earlier than the age of 50.

3. Abnormal Bowel Habits: If you experience abnormal bowel habits, including persistent diarrhea, constipation, or rectal bleeding, you should speak to your doctor about the possibility of having a colonoscopy.

4. Unexplained Abdominal Pain: If you experience unexplained abdominal pain, bloating, or discomfort, a colonoscopy can help identify the cause of your symptoms.

5. Inflammatory Bowel Disease: If you have a history of inflammatory bowel disease, including Crohn's disease or ulcerative colitis, you may be at an increased risk of developing colorectal cancer. Colonoscopy is recommended for people with inflammatory bowel disease.

6. Follow-Up after Previous Polyps: If you have had polyps detected during a previous colonoscopy, your doctor may recommend follow-up colonoscopy to ensure that the polyps have not returned or developed into cancer.

7. Age 50 or Older: If you are aged 50 or older, you should speak to your doctor about the possibility of having a colonoscopy. Regular colonoscopy screenings can help detect and prevent colorectal cancer.

8. Virtual Colonoscopy not Possible: If virtual colonoscopy is not possible or not available, colonoscopy is the preferred screening test for colorectal cancer.

9. Higher Risk for Colorectal Cancer: If you have a higher risk of developing colorectal cancer due to factors such as family history, obesity, or smoking, your doctor may recommend earlier or more frequent colonoscopy screenings.

10. Health Insurance: Many health insurance plans cover colonoscopy as a preventive screening test, making it an accessible and affordable option for many people.

A colonoscopy is an essential screening tool for the early detection and prevention of colorectal cancer. If you are aged 50 or older, have a family history of colorectal cancer, or experience any gastrointestinal symptoms, talk to your doctor about the possibility of having a colonoscopy. Regular colonoscopy screenings can help detect and remove precancerous polyps before they develop into cancer, reducing the risk of developing colorectal cancer.

The Colon and Rectum

The colon and rectum are essential parts of the digestive system, responsible for the absorption of water and nutrients from the food we eat. These organs also play a crucial role in the elimination of waste from the body. However, the colon and rectum can also be the site of various diseases, including colorectal cancer, inflammatory bowel disease, diverticulitis, and other conditions that can cause abdominal pain, bloating, diarrhea, constipation, and other symptoms.

Colonoscopy is a medical procedure that allows doctors to examine the colon and rectum for any abnormalities, including polyps, inflammation, or other issues. The procedure is an essential tool for the early detection and prevention of colorectal cancer, the third most common cancer in the United States.

The Colon

The colon, also known as the large intestine, is a muscular tube that is approximately five to six feet long. The colon is divided into several segments, including the cecum, ascending colon, transverse colon, descending colon, sigmoid colon, and rectum.

The primary function of the colon is to absorb water and electrolytes from the undigested food that has passed through the small intestine. The colon also absorbs vitamins produced by the gut bacteria and helps to form solid feces, which are then stored in the rectum until they are eliminated from the body.

The Rectum

The rectum is the final portion of the large intestine and is approximately six to eight inches long. The rectum is located in the pelvis and is connected to the anus, which is the opening at the end of the digestive tract.

The primary function of the rectum is to store feces until they can be eliminated from the body through the anus. The rectum is lined with muscles that help to control the passage of feces out of the body.

Colonoscopy and the Colon and Rectum

Colonoscopy is a medical procedure that allows doctors to examine the inside of the colon and rectum for any abnormalities, including polyps, inflammation, or other issues. The procedure involves the use of a colonoscope, which is a long, flexible tube with a tiny camera and light attached to its tip.

During the colonoscopy procedure, the colonoscope is inserted through the anus and advanced slowly into the colon while inflating it with air to allow for a better view. The camera on the colonoscope transmits images of the inside of the colon to a monitor in the exam room, allowing the doctor to examine the lining of the colon for any abnormalities.

If the doctor finds any polyps during the examination, they may remove them using specialized tools inserted through the colonoscope. The removed polyps are then sent to a laboratory for further analysis to determine if they are cancerous or precancerous.

Colonoscopy is an essential screening tool for the early detection and prevention of colorectal cancer, which is the third most common cancer in the United States. According to the American Cancer Society, colorectal cancer is expected to cause over 52,000 deaths in the United States in 2021 alone.

Screening for colorectal cancer using colonoscopy is recommended for people aged 50 and above, or earlier if you have a family history of colorectal cancer, inflammatory bowel disease, or other risk factors. Regular colonoscopy screenings can help detect and remove precancerous polyps before they develop into cancer, reducing the risk of developing colorectal cancer.

In addition to screening for colorectal cancer, colonoscopy can also be used to investigate the cause of various gastrointestinal symptoms, such as abdominal pain, diarrhea, constipation, and rectal bleeding. Colonoscopy can help diagnose conditions such as inflammatory bowel disease, diverticulitis, and other gastrointestinal conditions.

Anatomy and Function

The colon and rectum are critical organs of the digestive system responsible for the elimination of waste and absorption of water and nutrients from the food we eat. Understanding the anatomy and function of these organs is essential for the early detection and prevention of diseases such as colorectal cancer, inflammatory bowel disease, and other gastrointestinal conditions.

Anatomy of the Colon and Rectum

The colon, also known as the large intestine, is a muscular tube that is approximately five to six feet long. The colon is divided into several segments, including the cecum, ascending colon, transverse colon, descending colon, sigmoid colon, and rectum.

The cecum is the beginning of the colon and is located in the lower right side of the abdomen. The ascending colon runs upward on the right side of the abdomen, and the transverse colon runs horizontally across the abdomen. The descending colon runs downward on the left side of the abdomen, and the sigmoid colon connects the descending colon to the rectum.

The rectum is the final portion of the large intestine and is approximately six to eight inches long. The rectum is located in the pelvis and is connected to the anus, which is the opening at the end of the digestive tract.

Function of the Colon and Rectum

The primary function of the colon is to absorb water and electrolytes from the undigested food that has passed through the small intestine. The colon also absorbs vitamins produced by the gut bacteria and helps to form solid feces, which are then stored in the rectum until they are eliminated from the body.

The rectum is responsible for storing feces until they can be eliminated from the body through the anus. The rectum is lined with muscles that help to control the passage of feces out of the body.

Colonoscopy and the Colon and Rectum

Colonoscopy is a medical procedure that allows doctors to examine the inside of the colon and rectum for any abnormalities, including polyps, inflammation, or other issues. The procedure involves the use of a colonoscope, which is a long, flexible tube with a tiny camera and light attached to its tip.

During the colonoscopy procedure, the colonoscope is inserted through the anus and advanced slowly into the colon while inflating it with air to allow for a better view. The camera on the colonoscope transmits images of the inside of the colon to a monitor in the exam room, allowing the doctor to examine the lining of the colon for any abnormalities.

If the doctor finds any polyps during the examination, they may remove them using specialized tools inserted through the colonoscope. The removed polyps are then sent to a laboratory for further analysis to determine if they are cancerous or precancerous.

Colonoscopy is an essential screening tool for the early detection and prevention of colorectal cancer, which is the third most common cancer in the United States. According to the American Cancer Society, colorectal cancer is expected to cause over 52,000 deaths in the United States in 2021 alone.

Screening for colorectal cancer using colonoscopy is recommended for people aged 50 and above, or earlier if you have a family history of colorectal cancer, inflammatory bowel disease, or other risk factors. Regular colonoscopy screenings can help detect and remove precancerous polyps before they develop into cancer, reducing the risk of developing colorectal cancer.

In addition to screening for colorectal cancer, colonoscopy can also be used to investigate the cause of various gastrointestinal symptoms, such as abdominal pain, diarrhea, constipation, and rectal bleeding. Colonoscopy can help diagnose conditions such as inflammatory bowel disease, diverticulitis, and other gastrointestinal conditions.

Common Diseases and Conditions

The colon and rectum are vital organs of the digestive system responsible for the absorption of water and nutrients from the food we eat and the elimination of waste from the body. Unfortunately, these organs can also be the site of various diseases and conditions that can cause abdominal pain, bloating, diarrhea, constipation, and other symptoms. Understanding the most common diseases and conditions of the colon and rectum is essential for the early detection and treatment of these conditions.

Colorectal Cancer

Colorectal cancer is the third most common cancer in the United States, with over 149,000 new cases diagnosed every year. The risk of developing colorectal cancer increases with age, with over 90% of cases occurring in people aged 50 and above. Other risk factors for colorectal cancer include a family history of the disease, a personal history of colorectal cancer or polyps, inflammatory bowel disease, and certain genetic conditions.

Colonoscopy is an essential screening tool for the early detection and prevention of colorectal cancer. Regular colonoscopy screenings can help detect and remove precancerous polyps before they develop into cancer, reducing the risk of developing colorectal cancer.

Inflammatory Bowel Disease

1. Inflammatory bowel disease (IBD) is a chronic condition that causes inflammation of the digestive tract, leading to symptoms such as abdominal pain, diarrhea, rectal bleeding, weight loss, and fatigue. There are two main types of IBD: Crohn's disease and ulcerative colitis.

Crohn's disease can affect any part of the digestive tract, from the mouth to the anus, and causes inflammation of the entire bowel wall. Ulcerative colitis, on the other hand, affects only the colon and rectum and causes inflammation and ulcers in the lining of the colon and rectum.

Colonoscopy is an essential tool for diagnosing and monitoring inflammatory bowel disease. The procedure can help detect inflammation, ulcers, and other abnormalities in the colon and rectum, allowing doctors to diagnose and treat the condition early.

Diverticulitis

Diverticulitis is a condition that occurs when small pouches or sacs, called diverticula, form in the lining of the colon and become inflamed or infected. The condition can cause symptoms such as abdominal pain, fever, nausea, vomiting, constipation, or diarrhea.

Diverticulitis is more common in older adults and can be caused by a low-fiber diet, lack of physical activity, obesity, smoking, or certain medications. Treatment for diverticulitis may include antibiotics, pain relief medication, and dietary changes.

Colonoscopy is not usually recommended during an acute episode of diverticulitis, but it may be necessary to rule out other conditions or to monitor the condition if it becomes chronic.

Hemorrhoids

Hemorrhoids are swollen veins in the anus or lower rectum that can cause pain, itching, bleeding, and discomfort. Hemorrhoids are more common in older adults, pregnant women, and people with chronic constipation or diarrhea.

Treatment for hemorrhoids may include over-the-counter creams and ointments, warm baths, and dietary changes. In severe cases, surgery may be necessary.

Colonoscopy is not usually necessary for the diagnosis or treatment of hemorrhoids, but it may be recommended if bleeding is persistent or if other conditions are suspected.

Indications for a Colonoscopy

Colonoscopy is a medical procedure that allows doctors to examine the colon and rectum for any abnormalities, including polyps, inflammation, or other issues. The procedure is an essential tool for the early detection and prevention of colorectal cancer, the third most common cancer in the United States. Here are some of the indications for getting a colonoscopy:

Screening for Colorectal Cancer

One of the primary indications for a colonoscopy is screening for colorectal cancer. The American Cancer Society recommends that people aged 45 and above undergo regular colonoscopy screenings for colorectal cancer, while the United States Preventive Services Task Force recommends screening for people aged 50 and above.

Regular colonoscopy screenings can help detect and remove precancerous polyps before they develop into cancer, reducing the risk of developing colorectal cancer. People with a family history of colorectal cancer, inflammatory bowel disease, or other risk factors may need to start screening earlier or undergo more frequent screenings.

Investigating Gastrointestinal Symptoms

Colonoscopy can also be used to investigate the cause of various gastrointestinal symptoms, such as abdominal pain, diarrhea, constipation, rectal bleeding, or unexplained weight loss. These symptoms may be signs of colorectal cancer or other gastrointestinal conditions that require further investigation.

Colonoscopy can help diagnose conditions such as inflammatory bowel disease, diverticulitis, and other gastrointestinal conditions that can cause these symptoms. It can also help rule out other conditions that may be causing the symptoms.

Monitoring for Recurrence of Colorectal Cancer

People who have had colorectal cancer in the past may need to undergo regular colonoscopy screenings to monitor for any signs of recurrence. Regular colonoscopy screenings can help detect any new polyps or tumors early, allowing for prompt treatment and better outcomes.

Monitoring for Polyps

People who have had polyps in the past may need to undergo regular colonoscopy screenings to monitor for any new polyps. Polyps are abnormal growths in the colon or rectum that can become cancerous if left untreated.

Removing polyps during a colonoscopy can help prevent colorectal cancer from developing. People with a history of polyps may need to undergo more frequent colonoscopy screenings than those without a history of polyps.

Follow-Up After Abnormal Results on Other Tests

People who have had abnormal results on other tests, such as a fecal occult blood test or a sigmoidoscopy, may need to undergo a colonoscopy to investigate further. These tests may have detected signs of colorectal cancer or other gastrointestinal conditions that require further investigation.

Screening for Colorectal Cancer

Colorectal cancer is the third most common cancer in the United States, with over 149,000 new cases diagnosed every year. The disease can be deadly if not detected and treated early. However, when detected early, the five-year survival rate for colorectal cancer is over 90%. One of the most effective ways to detect and prevent colorectal cancer is through regular colonoscopy screenings.

Screening Recommendations

The American Cancer Society recommends that people aged 45 and above undergo regular colonoscopy screenings for colorectal cancer. However, the United States Preventive Services Task Force recommends screening for people aged 50 and above.

People with a family history of colorectal cancer, inflammatory bowel disease, or other risk factors may need to start screening earlier or undergo more frequent screenings. Your doctor can help determine when you should start screening and how often you should undergo screening.

Preparing for a Colonoscopy

Before undergoing a colonoscopy, your doctor will give you specific instructions on how to prepare for the procedure. The preparation typically involves fasting for several hours before the procedure and taking a laxative or other medication to clean out the colon.

The laxative or other medication can cause diarrhea and cramping, so it is essential to stay close to a bathroom during the preparation process. It is also important to follow your doctor's instructions carefully to ensure that your colon is adequately cleaned out before the procedure.

The Procedure

During the colonoscopy procedure, you will be given anesthesia to help you relax and prevent pain. The doctor will insert a colonoscope, which is a long, flexible tube with a tiny camera and light attached to its tip, into the rectum and advance it slowly through the colon.

The camera on the colonoscope transmits images of the inside of the colon to a monitor in the exam room, allowing the doctor to examine the lining of the colon for any abnormalities, such as polyps or other growths. If the doctor finds any polyps during the examination, they may remove them using specialized tools inserted through the colonoscope.

The procedure typically takes about 30 minutes to an hour to complete, and most people can go home the same day. However, you may feel groggy or tired for a few hours after the procedure due to the effects of the anesthesia.

Risks and Side Effects

Like any medical procedure, colonoscopy carries some risks and side effects. The risks of colonoscopy include bleeding, infection, and perforation of the colon or rectum. However, these complications are rare, occurring in less than 1% of cases.

The most common side effects of colonoscopy are bloating, cramping, and gas. These side effects usually go away within a few hours after the procedure.

Benefits of Screening

Regular colonoscopy screenings can help detect and remove precancerous polyps before they develop into cancer, reducing the risk of developing colorectal cancer. In addition, colonoscopy can help diagnose and treat other gastrointestinal conditions, such as inflammatory bowel disease, diverticulitis, and other gastrointestinal conditions.

According to the American Cancer Society, people who undergo regular colonoscopy screenings have a 60% lower risk of dying from colorectal cancer than those who do not undergo screening.

Diagnosis of Gastrointestinal Symptoms

Gastrointestinal symptoms such as abdominal pain, bloating, diarrhea, constipation, and rectal bleeding can be signs of various conditions, including inflammatory bowel disease, diverticulitis, colorectal cancer, and other gastrointestinal disorders. Diagnosing the cause of these symptoms is essential for proper treatment, and one of the most effective diagnostic tools is colonoscopy.

What is Colonoscopy?

Colonoscopy is a medical procedure that allows doctors to examine the colon and rectum for any abnormalities, including polyps, inflammation, or other issues. During the procedure, the doctor inserts a colonoscope, a long, flexible tube with a tiny camera and light attached to its tip, into the rectum and advances it slowly through the colon.

The camera on the colonoscope transmits images of the inside of the colon to a monitor in the exam room, allowing the doctor to examine the lining of the colon for any abnormalities. If the doctor finds any polyps during the examination, they may remove them using specialized tools inserted through the colonoscope.

Colonoscopy can also be used to take tissue samples for biopsy, allowing doctors to examine the tissue under a microscope for signs of inflammation, infection, or cancer.

When is Colonoscopy Indicated?

Colonoscopy is indicated for a variety of gastrointestinal symptoms and conditions, including:

Investigating Abdominal Pain and Bloating

Abdominal pain and bloating can be signs of various gastrointestinal conditions, such as inflammatory bowel disease, diverticulitis, or colorectal cancer. Colonoscopy can help diagnose these conditions by allowing doctors to examine the lining of the colon and rectum for any abnormalities.

Screening for Colorectal Cancer

Regular colonoscopy screenings are recommended for people aged 45 and above to screen for colorectal cancer, the third most common cancer in the United States. People with a family history of colorectal cancer or other risk factors may need to start screening earlier or undergo more frequent screenings.

Investigating Rectal Bleeding

Rectal bleeding can be a sign of various gastrointestinal conditions, including hemorrhoids, diverticulitis, or colorectal cancer. Colonoscopy can help diagnose these conditions by allowing doctors to examine the lining of the colon and rectum for any abnormalities.

Monitoring for Recurrence of Colorectal Cancer

People who have had colorectal cancer in the past may need to undergo regular colonoscopy screenings to monitor for any signs of recurrence. Regular colonoscopy screenings can help detect any new polyps or tumors early, allowing for prompt treatment and better outcomes.

Monitoring for Polyps

People who have had polyps in the past may need to undergo regular colonoscopy screenings to monitor for any new polyps. Polyps are abnormal growths in the colon or rectum that can become cancerous if left untreated.

Removing polyps during a colonoscopy can help prevent colorectal cancer from developing. People with a history of polyps may need to undergo more frequent colonoscopy screenings than those without a history of polyps.

Monitoring Inflammatory Bowel Disease

Inflammatory bowel disease (IBD) is a chronic condition that affects the digestive system. The two most common types of IBD are Crohn's disease and ulcerative colitis. IBD can cause a variety of symptoms, including abdominal pain, diarrhea, and weight loss. While there is no cure for IBD, it can be managed with proper treatment, which may include medication, dietary changes, and in some cases, surgery. Regular monitoring of IBD is essential for ensuring that treatment is effective and that the disease is not progressing.

What is Monitoring for IBD?

Monitoring for IBD involves regular check-ups with a gastroenterologist or other healthcare provider who specializes in the treatment of IBD. During these check-ups, the provider will assess the patient's symptoms and perform various tests to evaluate the effectiveness of treatment and monitor the progression of the disease.

One of the most effective diagnostic tools for monitoring IBD is colonoscopy. During a colonoscopy, the doctor inserts a colonoscope, a long, flexible tube with a tiny camera and light attached to its tip, into the rectum and advances it slowly through the colon. The camera on the colonoscope transmits images of the inside of the colon to a monitor in the exam room, allowing the doctor to examine the lining of the colon for any abnormalities, such as inflammation, ulcers, or other signs of IBD.

In addition to colonoscopy, other tests may be used to monitor IBD, including blood tests, stool tests, and imaging studies, such as X-rays or CT scans.

When is Monitoring for IBD Indicated?

Monitoring for IBD is indicated for people who have been diagnosed with Crohn's disease or ulcerative colitis or who have symptoms that suggest IBD. Regular monitoring is essential for ensuring that treatment is effective and that the disease is not progressing.

People with IBD may need to undergo monitoring more frequently if they experience a flare-up of symptoms or if their treatment plan changes. Your healthcare provider can help determine how often you should undergo monitoring based on your individual needs and symptoms.

What are the Benefits of Monitoring for IBD?

Regular monitoring for IBD has several benefits, including:

1. Early detection of disease progression: Regular monitoring can help detect any changes in the disease that may indicate that it is progressing. Early detection allows for prompt treatment and better outcomes.

2. Evaluation of treatment effectiveness: Monitoring can help evaluate the effectiveness of the current treatment plan and determine whether adjustments are needed.

3. Identification of complications: IBD can cause various complications, such as strictures, abscesses, or fistulas. Monitoring can help detect these complications early, allowing for prompt treatment.

4. Prevention of colorectal cancer: People with IBD have an increased risk of developing colorectal cancer. Regular monitoring can help detect any precancerous changes in the colon, allowing for prompt treatment and prevention of cancer.

What are the benefits of a colonoscopy?

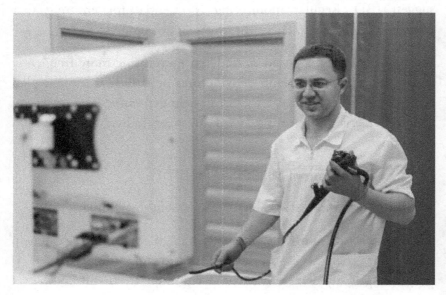

One of the main benefits of a colonoscopy is its ability to detect colon cancer at an early stage. Colon cancer is the third most common cancer in men and women in the United States and the second leading cause of cancer-related deaths. However, if caught early, the survival rate for colon cancer is over 90%. A colonoscopy can detect colon cancer before symptoms even appear, making it a crucial tool in the early detection and treatment of this disease.

A colonoscopy can also detect and remove precancerous polyps. Polyps are small growths that can form on the lining of the colon, and while not all polyps are cancerous, some can develop into cancer over time. During a colonoscopy, the doctor can identify and remove these polyps, preventing them from turning into cancer.

In addition to colon cancer and polyps, a colonoscopy can also detect and diagnose other conditions affecting the colon such as inflammatory bowel disease (IBD) and diverticulitis. IBD is a group of inflammatory conditions that affect the digestive system, including Crohn's disease and Ulcerative colitis. A colonoscopy can help diagnose these conditions and provide a starting point for treatment. Diverticulitis is a condition where small pouches form in the colon and can become infected or inflamed. A colonoscopy can help diagnose and monitor this condition.

A colonoscopy can also provide a more comprehensive evaluation of the colon than other screening tests such as fecal occult blood test (FOBT) or stool DNA test. These tests can only detect blood in the stool and abnormal cells respectively, but a colonoscopy allows the doctor to directly visualize the inside of the colon, providing a more detailed and accurate evaluation of the colon.

Another benefit of a colonoscopy is that it is a very safe procedure. Complications are rare, and the risk of a serious complication is less than 1 in 1,000. The procedure is performed while the patient is under sedation, which means they are awake but relaxed and comfortable. The procedure typically takes between 30 minutes to an hour, and the patient can go home the same day.

Colonoscopy is a well-established screening tool, and the American Cancer Society recommends that adults at average risk of colon cancer begin regular screening at age 45. For adults at high risk, such as those with a family history of colon cancer, screening may begin earlier. A colonoscopy is usually performed every 10 years for adults at average risk, and more frequently for those at high risk.

Screening Guidelines

Screening for colorectal cancer is an essential part of early detection and prevention of the disease. While colonoscopy is considered the gold standard for colorectal cancer screening, there are other screening options available. Here are the current screening guidelines for colorectal cancer:

Average-risk individuals

For individuals at average risk of developing colorectal cancer, the American Cancer Society recommends starting screening at age 45 with one of the following options:

Colonoscopy every 10 years

CT colonography (virtual colonoscopy) every 5 years

Flexible sigmoidoscopy every 5 years

Double-contrast barium enema every 5 years

Fecal immunochemical test (FIT) every year

Stool DNA test every 3 years

It's important to note that colonoscopy is the only screening option that can both detect and remove precancerous polyps.

High-risk individuals

For individuals with a family history of colorectal cancer or certain genetic conditions, screening should begin earlier and may be more frequent. Here are the recommended guidelines:

Individuals with a first-degree relative (parent, sibling, or child) diagnosed with colorectal cancer before age 60 should begin screening at age 40 or 10 years before the age at which the relative was diagnosed, whichever is earlier.

Individuals with a family history of a hereditary colorectal cancer syndrome should begin screening at an earlier age and may require more frequent screening. Examples of hereditary colorectal cancer syndromes include Lynch syndrome and familial adenomatous polyposis (FAP).

Individuals with a history of precancerous polyps or colorectal cancer

For individuals with a history of precancerous polyps or colorectal cancer, follow-up screening may be necessary. Here are the recommended guidelines:

Individuals with a history of adenomatous polyps (precancerous polyps) should undergo a colonoscopy within 3 to 5 years after the initial polyp removal. The timing of subsequent colonoscopies will depend on the number, size, and location of polyps.

Individuals with a history of colorectal cancer should undergo a colonoscopy within 1 year after the initial diagnosis and treatment. The timing of subsequent colonoscopies will depend on the stage of the cancer and the patient's individual risk factors.

Screening cessation

For individuals at average risk who have a negative colonoscopy result, screening should be repeated every 10 years. However, if polyps are found during the colonoscopy, the follow-up screening interval may be shorter. For individuals at high risk, screening should continue at shorter intervals and may not stop.

Risk Factors for Colorectal Cancer

Colorectal cancer is the third most common cancer in the world, with an estimated 1.9 million new cases diagnosed in 2020. While the causes of colorectal cancer are not fully understood, there are several risk factors that can increase the likelihood of developing the disease. Here are some of the most common risk factors for colorectal cancer:

Age

The risk of developing colorectal cancer increases with age. Most cases of colorectal cancer occur in individuals over the age of 50, and the risk continues to increase as a person gets older.

Family history

Having a family history of colorectal cancer can increase the risk of developing the disease. Individuals with a first-degree relative (parent, sibling, or child) who has had colorectal cancer are at higher risk, especially if the relative was diagnosed at a young age.

Inherited genetic conditions

Certain genetic conditions can increase the risk of developing colorectal cancer. These include Lynch syndrome, familial adenomatous polyposis (FAP), and MUTYH-associated polyposis (MAP).

Personal history of precancerous polyps or colorectal cancer

Individuals who have had precancerous polyps (adenomas) or colorectal cancer in the past are at higher risk of developing the disease again.

Inflammatory bowel disease

Inflammatory bowel disease (IBD), including ulcerative colitis and Crohn's disease, can increase the risk of developing colorectal cancer, especially if the disease has been present for a long time.

Diet

A diet high in red and processed meats, as well as low in fruits, vegetables, and whole grains, can increase the risk of developing colorectal cancer.

Lifestyle factors

Several lifestyle factors can increase the risk of developing colorectal cancer, including smoking, heavy alcohol use, and physical inactivity.

Race and ethnicity

African Americans have a higher incidence and mortality rate of colorectal cancer than other racial and ethnic groups in the United States. The reasons for this are not fully understood, but may be related to differences in access to healthcare, diet, and other lifestyle factors.

Type 2 diabetes

Individuals with type 2 diabetes are at higher risk of developing colorectal cancer, although the reasons for this are not fully understood.

Prevention Strategies

Colorectal cancer is a preventable disease. While some risk factors, such as age and family history, cannot be changed, there are several prevention strategies that can reduce the risk of developing colorectal cancer. Here are some of the most effective prevention strategies:

Screening

Screening for colorectal cancer is essential for early detection and prevention of the disease. The gold standard for colorectal cancer screening is colonoscopy, which can both detect and remove precancerous polyps before they turn into cancer. Other screening options include stool-based tests, such as fecal immunochemical tests (FIT) and stool DNA tests, as well as imaging tests, such as CT colonography (virtual colonoscopy). It's important to discuss the best screening option with your healthcare provider and to follow the recommended screening guidelines.

Diet and exercise

A healthy diet and regular exercise can reduce the risk of developing colorectal cancer. A diet high in fruits, vegetables, and whole grains, and low in red and processed meats, can help prevent the disease. Regular exercise, such as brisk walking, can also reduce the risk of developing colorectal cancer.

Quit smoking

Smoking is a known risk factor for many types of cancer, including colorectal cancer. Quitting smoking can reduce the risk of developing the disease.

Limit alcohol consumption

Heavy alcohol use can increase the risk of developing colorectal cancer. Limiting alcohol consumption to moderate levels (up to one drink per day for women and up to two drinks per day for men) can help prevent the disease.

Maintain a healthy weight

Being overweight or obese can increase the risk of developing colorectal cancer. Maintaining a healthy weight through a healthy diet and regular exercise can help prevent the disease.

Reduce exposure to environmental toxins

Exposure to certain environmental toxins, such as asbestos and benzene, can increase the risk of developing colorectal cancer. Reducing exposure to these toxins can help prevent the disease.

Treat inflammatory bowel disease

Inflammatory bowel disease (IBD), including ulcerative colitis and Crohn's disease, can increase the risk of developing colorectal cancer. Treating IBD and maintaining regular follow-up care with a healthcare provider can help prevent the disease.

How is a colonoscopy performed?

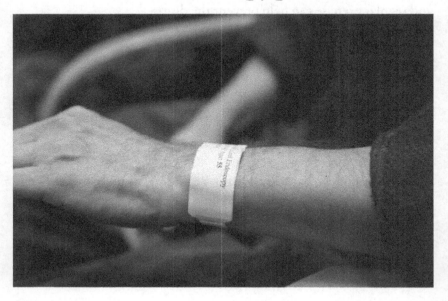

A colonoscopy is a medical procedure in which a doctor uses a thin, flexible tube with a camera at the end, called a colonoscope, to examine the inside of the colon and rectum. The procedure is usually performed as an outpatient procedure and typically takes between 30 minutes and an hour to complete.

Before the procedure, the patient will need to prepare by following a specific diet and taking a laxative or enema to clear the colon of feces. This is important to ensure a clear view of the inside of the colon during the procedure. The patient will also be asked to fast for several hours prior to the procedure.

On the day of the procedure, the patient will be given a sedative to help them relax and prevent discomfort during the procedure. This sedative is administered through an IV, and the patient will be awake during the procedure but will feel drowsy and relaxed.

The colonoscope is inserted into the rectum and advanced through the colon, while the doctor uses the camera to view the inside of the colon and rectum on a monitor. Air is also introduced into the colon through the colonoscope to help the doctor view the entire colon. The procedure is not usually painful, but some patients may experience some mild cramping or discomfort.

During the procedure, the doctor may remove small growths called polyps or take small samples of tissue (biopsies) for further analysis. If a polyp is found, it can be removed during the procedure using a special instrument passed through the colonoscope. This is known as a polypectomy.

After the procedure, the patient will be monitored for a short period of time until the sedative has worn off. The patient may feel some mild cramping or bloating for a short time after the procedure. The patient will be given instructions on how to resume normal activities and how to manage any discomfort.

It is important to note that the patient will not be able to drive after the procedure due to the sedative, so it is essential to arrange for someone to drive the patient home. The patient should also avoid making any important decisions or signing any legal documents for the rest of the day.

The results of the colonoscopy will be discussed with the patient by the doctor who performed the procedure. If polyps or tissue samples were taken, the results of any biopsies will be discussed with the patient at a later time.

Overall, a colonoscopy is a relatively safe and well-tolerated procedure that can help detect and diagnose a variety of conditions and diseases affecting the large intestine. The procedure is usually performed as an outpatient procedure and typically takes between 30 minutes and an hour to complete. It is important to follow the preparation instructions and aftercare instructions provided by the doctor to ensure a safe and successful procedure.

The Colonoscopy Procedure

A colonoscopy is a medical procedure used to examine the inside of the colon for any abnormalities, such as polyps or inflammation. Here's what you can expect during the colonoscopy procedure:

Preparation

Before the procedure, you will need to undergo bowel preparation to clean out your colon. This may involve drinking a bowel preparation solution and following a special diet.

You may also need to fast for a certain period before the procedure to ensure that your stomach is empty.

Anesthesia

During the procedure, you will receive sedation or anesthesia to help you relax and feel more comfortable. You may be conscious but drowsy or asleep during the procedure, depending on the type of sedation or anesthesia used.

Insertion of Colonoscope

The colonoscope is a long, flexible tube with a camera and light at the end. It is inserted into your rectum and slowly advanced through your colon.

As the colonoscope is advanced, the doctor will inflate your colon with air to help provide a clear view of the colon's lining.

Examination of Colon

As the colonoscope is advanced through your colon, the doctor will examine the lining of your colon for any abnormalities, such as polyps or inflammation.

If any abnormalities are found, the doctor may remove them during the procedure for further examination or biopsy.

Removal of Colonoscope

Once the colon has been fully examined, the colonoscope is slowly withdrawn from your colon.

Recovery

After the procedure, you will need to remain under observation for a period to ensure that you are recovering properly from the sedation or anesthesia.

You will also receive instructions on how to care for yourself after the procedure, including any restrictions on activity, diet, or medication.

Follow-Up

If any abnormalities were found during the procedure, you may need to undergo further testing or treatment, such as a biopsy or surgery.

You will also need to schedule follow-up appointments with your doctor to monitor your condition and ensure that you are recovering properly.

What happens during a colonoscopy?

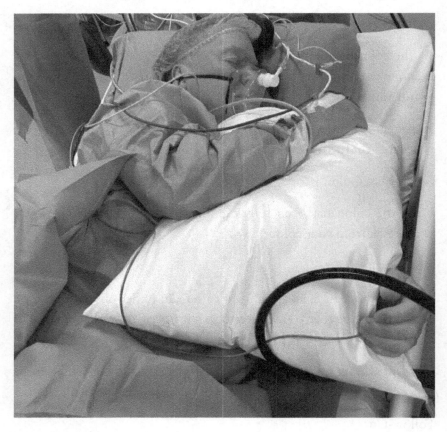

A colonoscopy is a medical procedure in which a doctor uses a thin, flexible tube with a camera at the end, called a colonoscope, to examine the inside of the colon and rectum. The procedure is typically performed as an outpatient procedure and typically takes between 30 minutes and an hour to complete.

Before the procedure, the patient will need to prepare by following a specific diet and taking a laxative or enema to clear the colon of feces. This is important to ensure a clear view of the inside of the colon during the procedure. The patient will also be asked to fast for several hours prior to the procedure.

On the day of the procedure, the patient will be asked to undress and will be given a gown to wear. An IV will be placed in the patient's arm to administer the sedative. The patient will be awake during the procedure but will feel drowsy and relaxed.

The colonoscope is inserted into the rectum and advanced through the colon, while the doctor uses the camera to view the inside of the colon and rectum on a monitor. Air is also introduced into the colon through the colonoscope to help the doctor view the entire colon. The procedure is not usually painful, but some patients may experience some mild cramping or discomfort.

As the colonoscope moves through the colon, the doctor will be able to see the inside of the colon and rectum. The doctor will be looking for any abnormal growths, such as polyps or tumors, as well as any signs of inflammation or bleeding. The doctor may also take small samples of tissue (biopsies) for further analysis. If a polyp is found, it can be removed during the procedure using a special instrument passed through the colonoscope. This is known as a polypectomy.

The colonoscope also has a small light and a camera on the end, which allows the doctor to see the inside of the colon and rectum in detail. The doctor will be able to see any abnormal growths, such as polyps or tumors, as well as any signs of inflammation or bleeding. The doctor may also take small samples of tissue (biopsies) for further analysis.

After the procedure, the patient will be moved to a recovery area where they will be monitored for a short period of time until the sedative has worn off. The patient may feel some mild cramping or bloating for a short time after the procedure. The patient will be given instructions on how to resume normal activities and how to manage any discomfort.

It is important to note that the patient will not be able to drive after the procedure due to the sedative, so it is essential to arrange for someone to drive the patient home. The patient should also avoid making any important decisions or signing any legal documents for the rest of the day.

The results of the colonoscopy will be discussed with the patient by the doctor who performed the procedure. If polyps or tissue samples were taken, the results of any biopsies will be discussed with the patient at a later time.

Overall, a colonoscopy is a relatively safe and well-tolerated procedure that can help detect and diagnose a variety of conditions and diseases affecting the large intestine. The procedure involves the insertion of a thin and flexible tube with a camera on the end, into the rectum and moving it through the colon while the doctor examines the inside of the colon and rectum on a monitor, looking for any abnormal growths, such as polyps or tumors, as well as any signs of inflammation or bleeding. The procedure may also involve taking small samples of tissue (biopsies) for further analysis. The patient will be given sedative to help them relax.

Sedation and Anesthesia

During a colonoscopy, sedation or anesthesia is often used to help patients relax and feel more comfortable during the procedure. Here's what you need to know about sedation and anesthesia during a colonoscopy:

Types of Sedation/Anesthesia

There are different types of sedation or anesthesia that may be used during a colonoscopy, including:

1. Conscious sedation: This is the most commonly used type of sedation for a colonoscopy. Conscious sedation involves the use of medication to help you relax and feel drowsy, but you remain conscious and can respond to commands.

2. Deep sedation: Deep sedation involves the use of medication to make you almost completely unconscious. You will not be able to respond to commands during the procedure.

3. General anesthesia: General anesthesia involves the use of medication to make you completely unconscious. You will not be aware of anything during the procedure.

Risks and Side Effects

Sedation and anesthesia can pose certain risks and side effects, including:

Difficulty breathing

Low blood pressure

Nausea and vomiting

Allergic reaction to the medication

It is important to inform your doctor of any medical conditions or medications you are taking that may increase your risk of complications.

Monitoring During Sedation/Anesthesia

During the procedure, you will be monitored closely to ensure that you are safe and comfortable. This may include monitoring your heart rate, blood pressure, and oxygen levels.

Your doctor will adjust the level of sedation or anesthesia based on your individual needs and medical history.

Recovery After Sedation/Anesthesia

After the procedure, you will need to recover from the effects of the sedation or anesthesia. This may take several hours, depending on the type and amount of medication used.

You will need someone to drive you home and should avoid driving or operating machinery for at least 24 hours after the procedure.

Precautions and Contraindications

Sedation and anesthesia should be used with caution in people with certain medical conditions, such as sleep apnea, heart disease, or lung disease.

Certain medications may also interact with the sedation or anesthesia medication, so it is important to inform your doctor of all medications you are taking.

The Colonoscope

The colonoscope is a crucial tool in the diagnosis and treatment of various gastrointestinal disorders, including colon cancer. A colonoscope is a long, flexible tube with a camera and light at the end that allows doctors to examine the inside of the colon. Here's what you need to know about the colonoscope:

Types of Colonoscopes

There are different types of colonoscopes that may be used during a colonoscopy, including:

1. Standard colonoscope: This is the most commonly used type of colonoscope. It is a long, flexible tube that can be maneuvered through the colon to examine the lining.

2. Pediatric colonoscope: This is a smaller colonoscope designed for use in children.

3. Sigmoidoscope: This is a shorter, rigid scope used to examine only the lower part of the colon.

How the Colonoscope Works

The colonoscope is inserted into the rectum and slowly advanced through the colon. The camera and light at the end of the colonoscope allow doctors to view the inside of the colon on a monitor.

The colonoscope is maneuvered through the colon by the doctor, who uses controls on the outside of the scope to move it in different directions.

Advantages of the Colonoscope

The colonoscope has several advantages over other diagnostic tools, including:

It allows for direct visualization of the colon's lining, making it easier to detect abnormalities such as polyps or cancer.

It can be used to perform biopsies or remove polyps during the procedure, which can help diagnose or treat conditions.

It is less invasive than other diagnostic tools, such as barium enemas or CT scans.

Risks of the Colonoscope

The colonoscope is generally considered safe, but it can pose certain risks, including:

4. Perforation of the colon: This is a rare but serious complication that can occur when the colonoscope punctures the colon.

5. Bleeding: This is another rare but serious complication that can occur when a biopsy or polyp removal is performed during the procedure.

6. Adverse reaction to sedation or anesthesia: Sedation or anesthesia may be used during the procedure and can pose certain risks.

Care and Maintenance of the Colonoscope

The colonoscope is a delicate piece of equipment that requires proper care and maintenance to ensure its effectiveness and longevity. After each use, the colonoscope must be thoroughly cleaned and disinfected to prevent infection and maintain its function.

Navigating the Colon

Navigating the colon during a colonoscopy can be a challenging task for doctors, as the colon is a long, flexible organ with many curves and turns. Here's what you need to know about navigating the colon during a colonoscopy:

Anatomy of the Colon

The colon is a long, muscular tube that forms the final part of the digestive system. It is divided into several sections, including the ascending colon, transverse colon, descending colon, sigmoid colon, and rectum.

The colon is a highly flexible organ with many curves and turns, which can make it difficult to navigate during a colonoscopy.

Colonoscopy Techniques

There are several techniques that doctors may use to navigate the colon during a colonoscopy, including:

1. Retroflexion: This technique involves turning the colonoscope backward at the end of the colon to examine areas that may be difficult to see otherwise.

2. Looping: This technique involves forming a loop in the colonoscope to help maneuver it through the colon.

3. Straightening: This technique involves straightening out any curves in the colon by applying pressure to the colonoscope.

Challenges of Navigating the Colon

Navigating the colon during a colonoscopy can be challenging for several reasons, including:

The colon is a highly flexible organ with many curves and turns, which can make it difficult to navigate.

The colon may be obstructed by stool or gas, which can make it more difficult to maneuver the colonoscope.

Some areas of the colon may be difficult to see, such as the cecum, which is located at the beginning of the colon.

Risks of Navigating the Colon

Navigating the colon during a colonoscopy can pose certain risks, including:

4. Perforation of the colon: This is a rare but serious complication that can occur when the colonoscope punctures the colon.

5. Bleeding: This is another rare but serious complication that can occur when a biopsy or polyp removal is performed during the procedure.

6. Adverse reaction to sedation or anesthesia: Sedation or anesthesia may be used during the procedure and can pose certain risks.

Importance of Proper Colon Navigation

Proper navigation of the colon during a colonoscopy is crucial for the accurate diagnosis and treatment of gastrointestinal disorders, including colon cancer.

If the colon is not properly navigated, abnormalities such as polyps or cancer may be missed, which can lead to delayed diagnosis and treatment.

Polyp Detection and Removal

Polyps are abnormal growths of tissue that can develop in the colon. Polyps are not usually cancerous, but some can develop into colon cancer if left untreated. During a colonoscopy, polyps can be detected and removed to prevent the development of colon cancer. Here's what you need to know about polyp detection and removal during a colonoscopy:

Polyp Detection

During a colonoscopy, the doctor uses the colonoscope to examine the inside of the colon for polyps. The colonoscope is equipped with a camera and light, which allows the doctor to visualize the lining of the colon and identify any abnormalities.

Polyps may appear as small, raised bumps or growths on the lining of the colon. The doctor may use a special tool to remove the polyp for further examination.

Polyp Removal

Polyp removal is typically performed during the colonoscopy. The doctor may use a special tool to remove the polyp, such as a wire loop or snare, which is used to cut the polyp from the colon wall.

After the polyp is removed, it is sent to a lab for further examination to determine if it is cancerous or not.

Benefits of Polyp Removal

The removal of polyps during a colonoscopy can have several benefits, including:

1. Early detection and prevention of colon cancer: Polyps can develop into colon cancer if left untreated, so the removal of polyps can prevent the development of colon cancer.

2. Improved survival rates: If colon cancer is detected early, the survival rate is much higher.

3. Improved quality of life: The removal of polyps can prevent the need for more invasive treatments, such as surgery or chemotherapy.

Risks of Polyp Removal

Polyp removal during a colonoscopy can pose certain risks, including:

4. Bleeding: The removal of a polyp can cause bleeding in the colon, which may require additional treatment.

5. Perforation of the colon: This is a rare but serious complication that can occur when the colonoscope punctures the colon during the polyp removal.

6. Adverse reaction to sedation or anesthesia: Sedation or anesthesia may be used during the procedure and can pose certain risks.

Follow-Up Care

After a colonoscopy, it is important to follow-up with your doctor for further care. If polyps were removed, your doctor may recommend more frequent colonoscopies to monitor for the development of new polyps.

It is also important to maintain a healthy lifestyle, including a balanced diet, regular exercise, and avoidance of smoking and excessive alcohol consumption, to reduce the risk of developing colon cancer.

Types of Polyps

Polyps are abnormal growths of tissue that can develop in the colon. There are several types of polyps that can develop, and each type has different characteristics and risks. Here's what you need to know about the types of polyps that can be detected during a colonoscopy:

Adenomatous Polyps

Adenomatous polyps are the most common type of polyp that can develop in the colon. These polyps are usually benign, but some can develop into colon cancer if left untreated.

Adenomatous polyps can be further classified as:

1. Tubular adenomas: These polyps are small and have a long, narrow shape.

2. Villous adenomas: These polyps are large and have a flat, finger-like shape.

3. Tubulovillous adenomas: These polyps have a combination of both tubular and villous features.

Hyperplastic Polyps

Hyperplastic polyps are the most common type of polyp that is found in the colon. These polyps are usually benign and do not have a significant risk of developing into colon cancer.

Hyperplastic polyps are usually small and have a round or oval shape.

Inflammatory Polyps

Inflammatory polyps are a type of polyp that can develop as a result of inflammation in the colon, such as in cases of inflammatory bowel disease (IBD).

These polyps are usually benign and do not have a significant risk of developing into colon cancer.

Inflammatory polyps are usually small and have a round or oval shape.

Juvenile Polyps

Juvenile polyps are a type of polyp that can develop in children. These polyps are usually benign and do not have a significant risk of developing into colon cancer.

Juvenile polyps can be further classified as:

4. Solitary juvenile polyps: These polyps occur as a single growth in the colon.

5. Multiple juvenile polyps: These polyps occur as multiple growths in the colon and are usually associated with a condition called juvenile polyposis syndrome.

Peutz-Jeghers Polyps

Peutz-Jeghers polyps are a type of polyp that can develop in the colon and other parts of the digestive system, such as the stomach and small intestine.

These polyps are usually benign but can increase the risk of developing other types of cancer, such as breast, ovarian, and pancreatic cancer.

Peutz-Jeghers polyps are usually small and have a round or oval shape, with a characteristic dark pigmentation.

Polypectomy Techniques

Polypectomy is the removal of polyps from the colon during a colonoscopy. There are several techniques that can be used to remove polyps, depending on the size and location of the polyp. Here's what you need to know about the different polypectomy techniques that can be used during a colonoscopy:

Snare Polypectomy

Snare polypectomy is the most common technique used to remove polyps during a colonoscopy. This technique involves using a wire loop called a snare to cut the polyp from the colon wall.

The snare is placed around the base of the polyp and tightened, cutting the polyp off from the colon wall. The snare is then removed along with the polyp.

Hot Biopsy Polypectomy

Hot biopsy polypectomy is a technique used to remove small polyps that are less than 5 mm in size. This technique involves using a small wire loop to cut the polyp from the colon wall, followed by the application of heat to the base of the polyp to seal the area and prevent bleeding.

Hot biopsy polypectomy is usually performed on polyps that are considered low-risk for cancer.

Cold Snare Polypectomy

Cold snare polypectomy is a technique used to remove small polyps that are less than 10 mm in size. This technique involves using a wire loop to cut the polyp from the colon wall without the use of heat.

Cold snare polypectomy is a safe and effective technique for removing small polyps and is associated with a lower risk of bleeding compared to other techniques.

Endoscopic Mucosal Resection (EMR)

Endoscopic mucosal resection (EMR) is a technique used to remove larger polyps that cannot be removed with other techniques. This technique involves injecting a solution beneath the polyp to raise it from the colon wall, followed by the use of a snare or other cutting device to remove the polyp.

EMR is a more complex procedure than other polypectomy techniques and is typically performed by a gastroenterologist with specialized training.

Submucosal Injection

Submucosal injection is a technique used to remove larger polyps that are difficult to remove with other techniques. This technique involves injecting a solution beneath the polyp to lift it from the colon wall, allowing for easier removal.

Submucosal injection is typically performed in combination with other polypectomy techniques, such as snare polypectomy or EMR.

Importance of Polyp Removal

Polyps are abnormal growths of tissue that can develop in the colon. While some polyps are benign and do not pose a significant health risk, others can develop into colon cancer if left untreated. That's why it's important to remove polyps when they are detected during a colonoscopy. Here's what you need to know about the importance of polyp removal:

Polyps can develop into colon cancer

Polyps that are left untreated can develop into colon cancer over time. The risk of cancer increases with the size and number of polyps present in the colon. That's why it's important to remove polyps as soon as they are detected during a colonoscopy.

Early detection and treatment can prevent colon cancer

Colon cancer is highly treatable when detected early. By removing polyps during a colonoscopy, gastroenterologists can detect and treat colon cancer in its early stages, when it is most treatable.

Regular colonoscopies can prevent colon cancer

Regular colonoscopies are the best way to prevent colon cancer. By detecting and removing polyps before they have the chance to develop into cancer, patients can significantly reduce their risk of developing colon cancer.

Polyp removal is safe and effective

Polyp removal during a colonoscopy is a safe and effective procedure. Most polyps can be removed using a snare polypectomy technique, which involves cutting the polyp from the colon wall with a wire loop. This technique is associated with a low risk of complications and is highly effective for the removal of most polyps.

Patients may need follow-up colonoscopies

Patients who have polyps removed during a colonoscopy may need to undergo follow-up colonoscopies to monitor for the development of new polyps. The frequency of follow-up colonoscopies depends on the size and number of polyps that were removed, as well as the patient's individual risk factors for colon cancer.

Polyp removal can improve quality of life

Removing polyps during a colonoscopy can improve a patient's quality of life by reducing the risk of developing colon cancer. Patients who undergo regular colonoscopies and have polyps removed are able to live healthier, more active lives without the fear of developing colon cancer.

Colonoscopy and Colorectal Cancer Prevention

Colorectal cancer is one of the most common types of cancer in the United States. It's estimated that approximately 1 in 23 men and 1 in 25 women will develop colorectal cancer at some point in their lives. However, with the proper screening and prevention methods, colorectal cancer can be detected and treated early, improving the chances of survival. One of the most effective methods for colorectal cancer prevention is colonoscopy. Here's what you need to know about the relationship between colonoscopy and colorectal cancer prevention:

Colonoscopy can detect precancerous polyps

Precancerous polyps are abnormal growths of tissue that can develop in the colon. If left untreated, some polyps can develop into cancer. However, by performing a colonoscopy, a gastroenterologist can detect and remove polyps before they have the chance to develop into cancer. This is why it's important to undergo regular colonoscopies, especially as you get older.

Colonoscopy is highly effective at preventing colorectal cancer

Colonoscopy is the gold standard for colorectal cancer prevention. In fact, studies have shown that colonoscopy can reduce the risk of developing colorectal cancer by up to 80 percent. This is because the removal of precancerous polyps during a colonoscopy can prevent cancer from developing in the first place.

Colonoscopy is recommended for average-risk individuals starting at age 45

The American Cancer Society recommends that individuals at average risk for colorectal cancer undergo a colonoscopy starting at age 45. This is because the risk of developing colorectal cancer increases with age, and colonoscopy is an effective way to detect and prevent the development of the disease.

Patients with a family history of colorectal cancer may need earlier or more frequent colonoscopies

Patients with a family history of colorectal cancer may need to undergo colonoscopies earlier or more frequently than those at average risk. This is because having a family history of the disease increases the likelihood of developing colorectal cancer.

Other screening methods are available, but colonoscopy is the most effective

While other screening methods for colorectal cancer, such as stool tests and flexible sigmoidoscopy, are available, colonoscopy is the most effective method for preventing the development of the disease. This is because colonoscopy allows for the detection and removal of precancerous polyps, while other methods may only detect the presence of cancer after it has already developed.

Colonoscopy is a safe and well-tolerated procedure

Colonoscopy is a safe and well-tolerated procedure, with a low risk of complications. Most patients are sedated during the procedure and experience little to no discomfort. After the procedure, patients are typically able to resume their normal activities within a day or two.

Pediatric Colonoscopy Procedure

A colonoscopy is a medical procedure used to examine the inside of the colon and rectum, also known as the large intestine, for abnormalities or diseases. It is a common procedure used in adults to detect colon cancer, but it is also used in pediatric patients for various indications. Below we will discuss the indications for a pediatric colonoscopy, the preparation needed for the procedure, and the procedure itself.

Indications for a Pediatric Colonoscopy:

There are several indications for a pediatric colonoscopy, including:

1. Abdominal Pain: Recurring or chronic abdominal pain that is not responding to treatment may require a colonoscopy to determine the cause.

2. Diarrhea: Chronic or bloody diarrhea may require a colonoscopy to examine the colon for inflammation, infection, or other causes.

3. Constipation: Chronic constipation or obstipation (a condition where the colon becomes completely blocked) may require a colonoscopy to identify any anatomical or functional abnormalities.

4. Unexplained Weight Loss: Unexplained weight loss can be a symptom of various gastrointestinal disorders and may require a colonoscopy to identify the cause.

5. Rectal Bleeding: Bright red blood in the stool or rectal bleeding may require a colonoscopy to identify the source of the bleeding.

6. Family History: Children with a family history of colon cancer or polyps may require a colonoscopy as a preventative measure.

Preparation for a Pediatric Colonoscopy:

The preparation for a pediatric colonoscopy is similar to that of an adult colonoscopy. The patient will need to have a clear liquid diet for at least 24 hours before the procedure, and will need to take laxatives or other bowel-cleansing agents to empty the colon of all stool. The child may also be given antibiotics to reduce the risk of infection.

It is important for parents to discuss the procedure with their child beforehand and to answer any questions they may have. It may also be helpful to explain the importance of the procedure and what to expect during and after the procedure.

Procedure for a Pediatric Colonoscopy:

During the procedure, the child is placed under sedation to minimize discomfort and ensure cooperation. The procedure itself is similar to an adult colonoscopy, where a flexible tube with a camera is inserted into the rectum and guided through the colon to examine the tissue lining.

The pediatric colonoscope is typically smaller than the adult colonoscope to accommodate the smaller size of the child's colon. The procedure typically lasts between 30 minutes to an hour, depending on the findings and whether any biopsies or polyps need to be removed.

After the procedure, the child will need to rest for a period of time until the effects of the sedation have worn off. The child may also experience some discomfort, cramping, or bloating, but this usually subsides within a few hours.

In some cases, if biopsies or polyps were removed during the procedure, the child may need to be monitored for a short period of time for any signs of bleeding or infection. The results of the procedure will be discussed with the parents or guardians, and any necessary follow-up appointments or treatment plans will be made.

Post-Procedural Care

Post-Procedural Care after a Pediatric Colonoscopy

A pediatric colonoscopy is a medical procedure that allows a physician to examine the lining of a child's large intestine or colon using a flexible tube with a camera and light source. It is used to diagnose and treat a variety of conditions, including gastrointestinal bleeding, inflammatory bowel disease, and polyps. After the procedure, it is important for parents and caregivers to provide appropriate post-procedural care to ensure that the child recovers well and without any complications. Below we will discuss the post-procedural care for a pediatric colonoscopy.

Recovery Room

After the colonoscopy, the child will be taken to a recovery room where they will be closely monitored for about an hour. During this time, the child will be awake but may feel groggy or dizzy due to the sedative medications used during the procedure. The child's vital signs, such as heart rate, blood pressure, and oxygen levels, will be monitored to ensure that they are stable.

The child may experience some abdominal discomfort or bloating, which is normal after a colonoscopy. The medical staff will provide the child with pain medications as needed. Parents or caregivers are allowed to be with the child during this time.

Diet and Fluids

After the child has fully recovered from the sedative medications, they will be allowed to drink clear liquids, such as water, broth, apple juice, or popsicles. It is important to start with small sips and gradually increase the amount of fluids. The child should avoid drinking carbonated drinks, caffeine, and milk products for the first few hours after the procedure.

If the child tolerates clear liquids well, they may be allowed to eat soft foods, such as crackers, soup, or mashed potatoes, later on. It is important to avoid foods that are spicy, fatty, or high in fiber as they can cause discomfort or bowel irritation.

Activity Level

After a pediatric colonoscopy, the child should rest for the remainder of the day. The child should avoid any strenuous physical activities or exercise for at least 24 hours. The physician will provide specific instructions on when the child can resume their normal activities based on the findings during the procedure.

Follow-up Care

The physician will discuss the results of the colonoscopy with the parents or caregivers after the procedure. If any polyps or abnormal tissue were found during the colonoscopy, a biopsy may have been taken for further analysis. The physician will discuss any necessary follow-up procedures or treatments with the parents or caregivers.

It is important to closely monitor the child's condition for the first few days after the procedure. Parents or caregivers should watch for any signs of complications, such as severe abdominal pain, fever, or rectal bleeding, and report them to the physician immediately.

Colonoscopy in the Elderly

Colonoscopy is a procedure used to diagnose and treat various gastrointestinal diseases and conditions. While it is generally considered a safe and effective procedure for people of all ages, there are some special considerations when it comes to colonoscopy in the elderly population.

As people age, they may develop a higher risk of certain gastrointestinal diseases and conditions, such as colorectal cancer, inflammatory bowel disease, and diverticulitis. This is why regular screening and surveillance are recommended for individuals over the age of 50, or for those with a family history of colorectal cancer or other related conditions.

However, some elderly patients may be at a higher risk for complications related to colonoscopy. This is because they may have other underlying health conditions, such as heart disease, lung disease, or diabetes, that can make them more susceptible to anesthesia-related complications or other risks associated with the procedure.

Additionally, some elderly patients may be taking certain medications that can increase the risk of bleeding or other complications during and after colonoscopy. These medications may include blood thinners, nonsteroidal anti-inflammatory drugs (NSAIDs), and certain herbal supplements.

Despite these potential risks, colonoscopy can still be a valuable tool for diagnosing and treating gastrointestinal conditions in the elderly population. In fact, early detection and treatment of these conditions can be particularly important for older adults, as they may have a harder time recovering from illness or injury than younger individuals.

When preparing for colonoscopy in the elderly, it is important to carefully consider the patient's individual health history and any underlying medical conditions. The healthcare provider may also want to consider ordering additional tests or evaluations to assess the patient's overall health status and determine the best course of action.

During the procedure itself, special care may need to be taken to ensure the patient's comfort and safety. For example, the healthcare provider may need to use a smaller colonoscope or adjust the dosage of anesthesia to minimize the risk of complications.

After the procedure, it is important to closely monitor the patient for any signs of complications or adverse reactions. This may include monitoring vital signs, checking for bleeding or other complications, and providing appropriate pain management and post-procedure care.

In some cases, the healthcare provider may also recommend follow-up colonoscopy at shorter intervals than what is typically recommended for younger individuals. This may be necessary to ensure that any abnormalities are detected and treated as early as possible, before they have a chance to progress and become more difficult to manage.

Adaptations for Older Patients

As individuals age, their bodies undergo changes that can impact their health and make certain medical procedures more challenging. Colonoscopy, a common screening test for colorectal cancer, is no exception. While colonoscopy is generally considered safe and effective, there are certain adaptations and considerations that may be necessary for older patients.

One of the main concerns with colonoscopy in older patients is the increased risk of complications. Older patients may be more likely to experience adverse events such as bleeding or perforation, particularly if they have pre-existing medical conditions or are taking certain medications. As a result, it is important for healthcare providers to carefully assess the risks and benefits of colonoscopy in older patients, and to take steps to minimize the risk of complications.

One adaptation that may be necessary for older patients undergoing colonoscopy is the use of sedation. While sedation is often used during colonoscopy to help patients relax and minimize discomfort, it may be particularly important for older patients who may be more sensitive to pain and discomfort. However, the use of sedation also carries risks, and healthcare providers must carefully evaluate each patient's individual health status and medication use before determining the appropriate level of sedation.

Another consideration for older patients undergoing colonoscopy is the preparation process. Older patients may have difficulty tolerating the bowel preparation solution, which is used to clean the colon prior to the procedure. In some cases, healthcare providers may need to adjust the dose or type of bowel preparation solution used to minimize discomfort and ensure that the colon is adequately cleaned.

Additionally, older patients may be more susceptible to dehydration or electrolyte imbalances during the bowel preparation process. As a result, healthcare providers may need to monitor older patients more closely during the preparation process and take steps to address any imbalances that occur.

Finally, healthcare providers must also take into account any pre-existing medical conditions that may impact the safety or effectiveness of colonoscopy in older patients. For example, older patients with heart disease may be at increased risk of complications during colonoscopy, and may require additional monitoring or interventions to ensure their safety.

Despite these challenges, colonoscopy remains an important screening tool for colorectal cancer in older patients. In fact, the American Cancer Society recommends that individuals at average risk of colorectal cancer begin regular screening at age 45, with continued screening every 10 years or more frequently if certain risk factors are present.

In addition to its role in cancer screening, colonoscopy can also be used to diagnose and treat a variety of other gastrointestinal conditions that are more common in older patients. For example, colonoscopy may be used to diagnose and treat inflammatory bowel disease or to remove polyps that can cause bleeding or other symptoms.

What are the risks and complications associated with a colonoscopy?

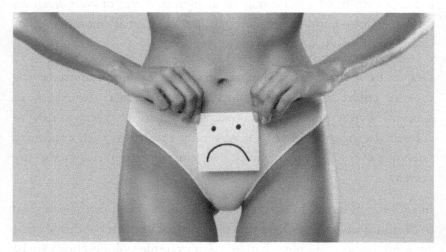

While colonoscopies are generally considered safe, there are certain risks and complications associated with the procedure. These include:

Perforation: The colonoscope can cause a small tear or hole in the colon, known as a perforation. This is a rare complication, occurring in less than 1% of cases, but can be serious if not treated promptly. Symptoms of a perforation may include severe abdominal pain, fever, and an abnormal heartbeat. Surgery may be required to repair the perforation.

Bleeding: Polyps or other abnormal growths in the colon may be removed during a colonoscopy, which can cause bleeding. This bleeding is usually mild and stops on its own, but in rare cases, a blood transfusion may be needed.

Infection: Any procedure that involves the insertion of a foreign object into the body carries a risk of infection. The risk of infection from a colonoscopy is low, but can be increased in people with weakened immune systems or other underlying medical conditions.

Anemia: Blood loss from a colonoscopy can lead to anemia, a condition characterized by a low red blood cell count. Anemia can cause symptoms such as fatigue, weakness, and pale skin.

Sedation complications: Colonoscopies are often performed with sedation to help the patient relax and be more comfortable during the procedure. Complications from sedation can include allergic reactions, breathing problems, and low blood pressure.

False positives and false negatives: A colonoscopy can miss small polyps or growths, leading to a false negative result. Additionally, a colonoscopy can sometimes detect polyps or growths that are not cancerous, leading to unnecessary follow-up tests and procedures.

Bowel preparation complications: Before a colonoscopy, the patient is typically asked to follow a special diet and take a laxative to clear the colon of feces. This bowel preparation can cause side effects such as dehydration, cramping, and diarrhea.

Long-term complications: In rare cases, a colonoscopy can lead to long-term complications such as bowel obstruction, chronic abdominal pain, and chronic diarrhea.

There is also a risk of bowel perforation, which can happen when the colonoscope is inserted into the colon. It is a rare complication, but if it occurs, it can be serious and require surgery.

Additionally, there is also a risk of bleeding after a colonoscopy. This can happen if a polyp is removed during the procedure or if the colonoscope causes an injury to the colon. The bleeding is usually mild and stops on its own, but in rare cases, a blood transfusion may be needed.

Some people may have an allergic reaction to the sedative used during the procedure. Symptoms of an allergic reaction can include hives, itching, and difficulty breathing.

A colonoscopy can also cause discomfort, such as cramping and bloating, for a few days after the procedure.

Overall, colonoscopies are considered safe and effective procedures, with a low risk of serious complications. However, as with any medical procedure, it is important for patients to understand the potential risks and discuss them with their doctor before deciding to undergo a colonoscopy.

Managing Complications

Colonoscopy is a safe and effective procedure for detecting and preventing colorectal cancer. However, as with any medical procedure, there is a risk of complications. Here are some of the most common complications of colonoscopy and how they can be managed:

Bleeding

Bleeding is a rare but possible complication of colonoscopy, especially if a polyp is removed. Most cases of bleeding are minor and can be managed with simple measures, such as applying pressure or using a special device to stop the bleeding. In rare cases, surgery may be necessary to stop the bleeding.

Perforation

Perforation, or a tear in the colon wall, is a rare but serious complication of colonoscopy. Perforation can occur if the colonoscope is passed too far into the colon or if a polyp is removed. Symptoms of perforation include severe abdominal pain, fever, and chills. Treatment for perforation may include surgery to repair the tear.

Adverse reaction to sedation

Sedation is commonly used during colonoscopy to help the patient relax and reduce discomfort. While sedation is generally safe, some individuals may have an adverse reaction, such as low blood pressure or difficulty breathing. These reactions can usually be managed with medication or by adjusting the level of sedation.

Infection

Infection is a rare complication of colonoscopy, but can occur if bacteria from the colon are introduced into the bloodstream during the procedure. Symptoms of infection may include fever, chills, and abdominal pain. Treatment for infection may include antibiotics.

Abdominal pain and bloating

Abdominal pain and bloating are common after colonoscopy, especially if a polyp is removed. These symptoms usually resolve within a few days, but can be managed with over-the-counter pain relievers and by drinking plenty of fluids.

Allergic reaction

Allergic reactions to the medications used during colonoscopy are rare but can occur. Symptoms of an allergic reaction may include hives, itching, and difficulty breathing. Treatment for an allergic reaction may include medication, such as antihistamines or epinephrine.

Missed polyps

While colonoscopy is a highly effective method for detecting and removing polyps, it is possible for some polyps to be missed. Factors that can increase the risk of missed polyps include the size and location of the polyp, as well as the experience of the colonoscopist. If a polyp is missed, it may continue to grow and become cancerous. For this reason, it's important to follow the recommended screening guidelines and to have regular follow-up colonoscopies as recommended by your healthcare provider.

Perforation

Perforation is a rare but serious complication of colonoscopy. It occurs when the colonoscope, the long, flexible tube used during the procedure, tears the colon wall. Perforation can cause severe abdominal pain and, if left untreated, can lead to life-threatening complications.

Causes of Perforation

Perforation can occur for several reasons, including:

1. Incorrect insertion technique: If the colonoscope is inserted too forcefully or at the wrong angle, it can cause a tear in the colon wall.

2. Polyp removal: Removing a polyp during colonoscopy increases the risk of perforation, especially if the polyp is large or located in a difficult-to-reach area.

3. Prior surgery: If the patient has had prior abdominal surgery, the risk of perforation may be higher due to adhesions or scar tissue.

4. Colon conditions: If the patient has a condition that affects the strength or integrity of the colon wall, such as diverticulitis or inflammatory bowel disease, the risk of perforation may be higher.

Symptoms of Perforation

The symptoms of perforation may include:

5. Severe abdominal pain: Perforation can cause sudden and severe abdominal pain that may be accompanied by nausea and vomiting.

6. Fever: If the colon wall is perforated, bacteria from the colon can enter the bloodstream and cause a fever.

7. Chills: The patient may experience chills or a feeling of coldness.

8. Rapid heartbeat: The heart may beat faster than normal due to the body's response to the infection.

9. Difficulty passing gas or stool: The patient may have difficulty passing gas or stool due to the tear in the colon wall.

Treatment of Perforation

If perforation is suspected during or after colonoscopy, immediate medical attention is necessary. Treatment for perforation may include:

10. Surgery: If the perforation is large or severe, surgery may be necessary to repair the tear in the colon wall.

11. Antibiotics: If there is an infection present, antibiotics may be prescribed to prevent further complications.

12. Monitoring: In some cases, the patient may be closely monitored in the hospital to ensure that the perforation does not worsen and that there are no further complications.

Prevention of Perforation

While perforation is a rare complication of colonoscopy, there are steps that can be taken to reduce the risk of perforation:

13. Choose an experienced colonoscopist: The risk of perforation is lower when the colonoscopy is performed by an experienced colonoscopist who is familiar with the procedure and knows how to minimize the risk of complications.

14. Follow the bowel preparation instructions: A thorough bowel preparation is necessary to ensure that the colon is clean and free of stool, which can obstruct the colonoscope and increase the risk of perforation.

15. Report any symptoms: If the patient experiences any symptoms after colonoscopy, such as severe abdominal pain or fever, it is important to report them to the healthcare provider immediately.

Bleeding

Bleeding is a common complication of colonoscopy. It occurs when the colonoscope, the long, flexible tube used during the procedure, causes a tear or injury to the colon wall, which can lead to bleeding. While bleeding after colonoscopy is usually mild and self-limited, in rare cases, it can be severe and require medical intervention.

Causes of Bleeding

Bleeding can occur during or after colonoscopy for several reasons, including:

1. Polyp removal: Removing a polyp during colonoscopy increases the risk of bleeding, especially if the polyp is large or located in a difficult-to-reach area.

2. Biopsy: If a biopsy is taken during colonoscopy, the area may bleed, especially if the biopsy is taken from a larger blood vessel.

3. Instrument trauma: If the colonoscope or other instruments used during colonoscopy cause injury to the colon wall, it can lead to bleeding.

4. Patient-related factors: Certain factors, such as blood-thinning medications, bleeding disorders, or diverticulosis, may increase the risk of bleeding after colonoscopy.

Symptoms of Bleeding

The symptoms of bleeding after colonoscopy may include:

5. Rectal bleeding: The patient may notice bright red blood in the stool or on the toilet paper.

6. Abdominal pain: If the bleeding is severe, the patient may experience abdominal pain or cramping.

7. Dizziness or weakness: If there is significant blood loss, the patient may experience dizziness or weakness.

8. Low blood pressure: In severe cases, the patient's blood pressure may drop due to significant blood loss.

Treatment of Bleeding

Most cases of bleeding after colonoscopy are mild and self-limited, and require no specific treatment. However, if the bleeding is severe or persistent, medical intervention may be necessary. Treatment for bleeding after colonoscopy may include:

9. Endoscopic intervention: If the bleeding is due to a polyp removal or other injury to the colon wall, endoscopic intervention may be necessary to stop the bleeding.

10. Blood transfusion: If the bleeding is severe and leads to significant blood loss, a blood transfusion may be necessary to replace the lost blood.

11. Medications: In some cases, medications may be used to help control bleeding, such as epinephrine injections or other vasoconstrictors.

Prevention of Bleeding

While bleeding is a potential complication of colonoscopy, there are steps that can be taken to reduce the risk of bleeding:

12. Choose an experienced colonoscopist: The risk of bleeding is lower when the colonoscopy is performed by an experienced colonoscopist who is familiar with the procedure and knows how to minimize the risk of complications.

13. Discontinue blood-thinning medications: If the patient is taking blood-thinning medications, they may need to be temporarily discontinued before the colonoscopy to reduce the risk of bleeding.

14. Report any symptoms: If the patient experiences any symptoms after colonoscopy, such as rectal bleeding or abdominal pain, it is important to report them to the healthcare provider immediately.

Post-Polypectomy Syndrome

Post-polypectomy syndrome (PPS) is a rare complication that can occur after a colonoscopy with polypectomy, which is the removal of a polyp from the colon. PPS is characterized by abdominal pain, fever, and sometimes rectal bleeding. While PPS is a rare complication, patients who undergo polypectomy should be aware of the signs and symptoms of PPS and should report any symptoms to their healthcare provider immediately.

Causes of Post-Polypectomy Syndrome

The exact cause of PPS is unknown, but it is thought to be related to a localized inflammatory response in the colon following polypectomy. The removal of a polyp can cause injury to the colon wall, which can lead to an inflammatory response. In some cases, this inflammatory response can be severe and result in PPS.

Symptoms of Post-Polypectomy Syndrome

The symptoms of PPS may include:

1. Abdominal pain: The patient may experience cramping or sharp pain in the abdomen, which can be severe.

2. Fever: The patient may develop a fever, which can be a sign of an infection.

3. Rectal bleeding: In some cases, PPS can cause rectal bleeding.

4. Nausea and vomiting: The patient may feel nauseous or vomit.

5. Diarrhea: The patient may have diarrhea, which can be watery or bloody.

Treatment of Post-Polypectomy Syndrome

The treatment of PPS depends on the severity of the symptoms. In most cases, the symptoms of PPS are mild and self-limited, and require no specific treatment. However, if the symptoms are severe, medical intervention may be necessary. Treatment for PPS may include:

6. Pain relief: The patient may be given pain medication to help relieve the abdominal pain.

7. Antibiotics: If the patient has a fever or other signs of infection, antibiotics may be necessary to treat the infection.

8. Fluids and electrolytes: If the patient is experiencing diarrhea or vomiting, they may need fluids and electrolytes to prevent dehydration.

9. Rest: The patient may need to rest and avoid strenuous activity until the symptoms subside.

Prevention of Post-Polypectomy Syndrome

While PPS is a rare complication, there are steps that can be taken to reduce the risk of developing PPS after polypectomy:

10. Choose an experienced colonoscopist: The risk of complications, including PPS, is lower when the colonoscopy is performed by an experienced colonoscopist who is familiar with the procedure and knows how to minimize the risk of complications.

11. Follow post-polypectomy instructions: After the polypectomy, the patient should follow the instructions given by the healthcare provider, including avoiding certain foods, medications, or activities for a period of time after the procedure.

12. Report any symptoms: If the patient experiences any symptoms after polypectomy, such as abdominal pain, fever, or rectal bleeding, it is important to report them to the healthcare provider immediately.

Colonoscopy and Cultural Considerations

Colonoscopy is a valuable diagnostic and preventive tool for detecting and preventing colorectal cancer. However, some individuals may have cultural or religious beliefs that impact their willingness to undergo the procedure. It is important for healthcare providers to understand and respect these beliefs while also educating patients on the benefits of colonoscopy.

One cultural consideration that may affect colonoscopy is the belief in modesty. Some cultures may view the procedure as invasive and uncomfortable, leading to reluctance or refusal to undergo the test. Providers can address this concern by explaining the procedure in detail, including how it is performed and what to expect during and after the procedure. Providers can also offer sedation to minimize discomfort and ensure the patient's privacy is respected throughout the procedure.

Religious beliefs may also impact a patient's decision to undergo colonoscopy. Some religious groups may view the procedure as unnecessary or contrary to their beliefs. Providers can address this concern by explaining the potential benefits of colonoscopy in preventing colorectal cancer and addressing any misconceptions the patient may have. Providers can also work with the patient to find alternatives to colonoscopy that align with their beliefs, such as fecal occult blood testing or stool DNA testing.

Language barriers may also impact a patient's understanding and willingness to undergo colonoscopy. Providers should strive to provide interpretation services or written materials in the patient's preferred language to ensure they have a complete understanding of the procedure and its benefits. Providers can also work with community organizations or cultural brokers to bridge communication gaps and address cultural considerations.

It is important for providers to approach cultural considerations with sensitivity and respect, taking into account the patient's beliefs and preferences. Providers should strive to provide patient-centered care that takes into account the patient's cultural background, beliefs, and values.

In addition to addressing cultural considerations, providers should also be aware of disparities in colonoscopy screening rates among certain populations. Studies have shown that individuals from racial and ethnic minority groups, as well as those with lower income and education levels, are less likely to undergo colonoscopy screening. Providers should work to identify and address these disparities through culturally tailored outreach and education efforts.

Finally, providers should also be aware of the role that family and community may play in a patient's decision to undergo colonoscopy. In some cultures, decision-making is a collective process that involves input from family members and trusted community members. Providers should work to engage with family members and community leaders to educate them on the benefits of colonoscopy and address any cultural considerations or concerns.

Cultural Barriers to Screening

Colonoscopy is a widely recommended screening tool for colorectal cancer. Despite the importance of early detection, cultural barriers to screening can hinder individuals from getting a colonoscopy. Cultural barriers can include language barriers, beliefs, and attitudes towards screening, and lack of knowledge about colorectal cancer and screening.

Language barriers are a common cultural barrier to screening. Individuals who speak a language other than English may struggle to communicate with their healthcare provider and understand the importance of getting a colonoscopy. Additionally, individuals who do not speak English may not have access to screening materials in their native language, further hindering their ability to receive proper screening.

Beliefs and attitudes towards screening can also be a cultural barrier to colonoscopy. Some individuals may hold beliefs that colonoscopy is unnecessary or uncomfortable, while others may feel uncomfortable discussing the topic with their healthcare provider. Cultural beliefs and attitudes can vary greatly between different ethnic and cultural groups, and it is important for healthcare providers to be sensitive to these beliefs and attitudes when discussing screening options.

Lack of knowledge about colorectal cancer and screening is another cultural barrier to colonoscopy. Many individuals from different cultural backgrounds may not have access to information about colorectal cancer and screening, or may not know where to find information. Additionally, some individuals may not know anyone who has had a colonoscopy and may be hesitant to undergo the procedure without knowing more about it.

To address cultural barriers to colonoscopy, healthcare providers should take steps to educate patients about the importance of screening, provide screening materials in multiple languages, and be sensitive to cultural beliefs and attitudes. Healthcare providers can also work with community leaders to promote colorectal cancer screening and provide educational resources to individuals in their community.

Another way to address cultural barriers to colonoscopy is to offer alternative screening methods, such as fecal occult blood tests or stool DNA tests, which do not require the same level of preparation or invasive procedure as a colonoscopy. These alternative methods may be more acceptable to individuals who are hesitant to undergo a colonoscopy.

In addition to addressing cultural barriers to screening, it is important to address disparities in colorectal cancer incidence and mortality rates among different ethnic and cultural groups. Some studies have shown that certain ethnic and cultural groups are more likely to develop colorectal cancer and less likely to receive screening, leading to higher mortality rates. To address these disparities, healthcare providers should work to increase awareness of colorectal cancer and screening among these groups, and provide targeted education and resources.

Addressing Disparities

Addressing Disparities: Ensuring Access to Colonoscopy for All

Colorectal cancer is the third most common cancer and the second leading cause of cancer-related deaths in the United States. The good news is that colorectal cancer is largely preventable with timely and regular screening, such as colonoscopy. However, disparities in screening rates exist among different populations, particularly among racial and ethnic minorities, low-income individuals, and those living in rural areas. These disparities have serious consequences, as individuals from these groups are more likely to be diagnosed with advanced-stage colorectal cancer and have worse outcomes. Addressing these disparities is crucial to reducing the burden of colorectal cancer, improving health equity, and saving lives.

Barriers to Screening

There are several barriers that contribute to disparities in colonoscopy screening rates. Lack of access to healthcare is a major barrier, particularly for uninsured or underinsured individuals who may not be able to afford the cost of the procedure. Even for those who have insurance, high deductibles or co-pays may deter them from getting screened. Language barriers and cultural beliefs may also prevent some individuals from seeking screening. Fear, anxiety, and embarrassment are common reasons why people avoid colonoscopy. In some cases, people may not have adequate knowledge about colorectal cancer and screening, which can lead to misconceptions and misinformation.

Strategies to Address Disparities

To address disparities in colonoscopy screening rates, it is important to implement strategies that target the specific barriers faced by different populations. Some of these strategies include:

2. Increasing access to healthcare: This can be achieved through expanding Medicaid coverage, providing subsidies or tax credits to help individuals purchase insurance, and creating more community health clinics in underserved areas.

3. Reducing the cost of colonoscopy: This can be done by implementing policies that require insurance companies to cover the full cost of screening, regardless of whether polyps are found or not. Additionally, offering free or low-cost screening programs can help to remove financial barriers.

4. Educating and raising awareness: This includes providing culturally appropriate educational materials in multiple languages and using community outreach to promote the importance of screening. Engaging primary care providers and other healthcare professionals to recommend screening to their patients can also increase awareness.

5. Addressing cultural beliefs and language barriers: It is important to provide culturally sensitive care and address any misconceptions or concerns that patients may have about the procedure. Providing interpretation services or using bilingual providers can help to overcome language barriers.

6. Improving patient experience: This includes ensuring that patients receive clear and comprehensive information about the procedure, providing comfortable and private facilities, and offering sedation options to alleviate anxiety and discomfort.

Culturally Competent Care

Cultural competence is a crucial aspect of healthcare that ensures that providers are respectful of and responsive to the unique cultural and linguistic needs of their patients. When it comes to colonoscopies, cultural competence is especially important given the many cultural barriers to screening that exist. Below we will explore what culturally competent care means in the context of colonoscopies and why it is important.

First, let's define what we mean by cultural competence. According to the National Institutes of Health (NIH), cultural competence is "the ability of individuals and systems to respond respectfully and effectively to people of all cultures, languages, classes, races, ethnic backgrounds, religions, and other diversity factors in a manner that recognizes, affirms, and values the worth of individuals, families, and communities, and protects and preserves the dignity of each." In other words, culturally competent care means understanding and respecting the unique cultural and linguistic needs of each patient and providing care that is tailored to those needs.

When it comes to colonoscopies, there are many cultural barriers to screening that can prevent patients from getting the care they need. For example, some cultures have taboos around discussing topics related to the colon or rectum, which can make it difficult to broach the subject of colonoscopies. Other cultures may view the healthcare system with suspicion or mistrust, making it difficult to convince patients to undergo screening. Still, others may not have access to healthcare due to economic or logistical barriers.

One way to address these cultural barriers is through culturally competent care. This means that providers take the time to understand the cultural and linguistic needs of their patients and tailor their approach accordingly. For example, a provider might take extra care to explain the colonoscopy procedure in a way that is culturally appropriate and sensitive. They might also provide written materials in the patient's preferred language or work with a medical interpreter to ensure that communication is clear and effective.

Another way to address cultural barriers to screening is through community outreach and education. By working with community leaders and organizations, healthcare providers can help to break down cultural taboos around colonoscopies and raise awareness about the importance of screening. They can also work to address economic and logistical barriers by providing free or low-cost screening options and helping patients navigate the healthcare system.

Ultimately, the goal of culturally competent care in the context of colonoscopies is to improve screening rates and reduce disparities in colon cancer outcomes. Studies have shown that patients who receive culturally competent care are more likely to participate in cancer screening programs and have better health outcomes overall. By taking the time to understand and respond to the unique cultural and linguistic needs of their patients, providers can help to ensure that all patients have access to the care they need to stay healthy.

How can I prepare for my colonoscopy?

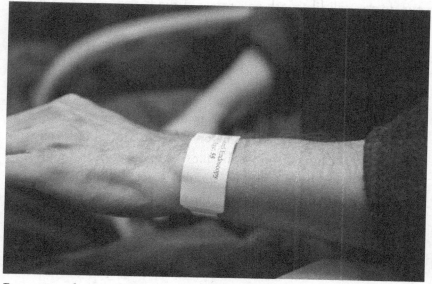

Preparing for a colonoscopy is an important step in ensuring a successful and comfortable procedure. The preparation process typically involves a combination of dietary changes, laxatives, and enemas to clean out the colon, making it easier for the doctor to view the inside of the colon during the procedure.

The first step in preparing for a colonoscopy is to schedule an appointment with your doctor to discuss the procedure and any specific instructions they may have. Your doctor will likely provide you with written instructions on how to prepare for the procedure, which you should carefully read and follow.

One of the most important parts of preparing for a colonoscopy is the dietary changes that will be required. A few days before the procedure, your doctor will likely ask you to avoid foods that can cause gas or discomfort such as beans, broccoli, cabbage, and certain fruits. You will also be asked to follow a low-fiber diet, which means avoiding foods that are high in fiber such as whole-grain breads, cereals, and fruits.

It is also important to avoid eating and drinking for a certain number of hours before the procedure. Your doctor will give you specific instructions on how long to fast before the procedure, but it is usually between 6 to 12 hours. You will be allowed to drink clear liquids such as water, tea, and broth, but you should avoid anything with red or purple color, as it can interfere with the view during the procedure.

In addition to dietary changes, you will also need to take laxatives to clean out the colon before the procedure. The most common laxatives used are polyethylene glycol (PEG) and sodium phosphate. These laxatives work by drawing water into the colon, which helps to soften and move the stool. It is important to follow the instructions on the package and the instructions given by your doctor carefully.

You may also be asked to use an enema to clean out the rectum, which is the last part of the colon the doctor will examine during the procedure. An enema is a liquid solution that is inserted into the rectum, which helps to flush out the rectum and lower colon.

It is also important to arrange for transportation home after the procedure as the sedation can affect your ability to drive or operate heavy machinery. It's also a good idea to have someone stay with you for the first 24 hours after the procedure, just in case you experience any complications.

The day before the procedure, it is important to follow the instructions given by your doctor regarding diet, laxatives and enemas. It is also important to follow any other instructions given by your doctor, such as what medications to take or avoid, and what to wear during the procedure.

It is normal to feel a bit anxious about the procedure, but it is important to remember that a colonoscopy is a very safe and common procedure that is performed millions of times each year. The preparation process can be uncomfortable, but it is a minor inconvenience for the peace of mind and early detection that the procedure can bring.

Preparing for a Colonoscopy

Colonoscopy is a medical procedure that allows doctors to examine the colon and rectum for any abnormalities, including polyps, inflammation, or other issues. Before undergoing a colonoscopy, it is essential to prepare your body adequately to ensure that the procedure is as safe and effective as possible.

Here are some tips for preparing for a colonoscopy:

Talk to Your Doctor

Before undergoing a colonoscopy, it is important to talk to your doctor about any medications you are taking, including over-the-counter medications, supplements, and vitamins. Some medications, such as blood thinners, may need to be stopped before the procedure.

You should also inform your doctor if you have any medical conditions, such as heart or lung disease, that may affect the procedure.

Follow the Pre-Procedure Diet

A few days before the colonoscopy, you will need to follow a pre-procedure diet. The purpose of the diet is to clear out your colon, allowing the doctor to examine the lining of the colon for any abnormalities.

The pre-procedure diet typically involves avoiding solid foods and drinking clear liquids, such as water, tea, and broth. You may also need to take laxatives or other medications to help clean out your colon.

It is important to follow the pre-procedure diet carefully to ensure that your colon is adequately cleaned out before the procedure.

Plan for the Day of the Procedure

On the day of the colonoscopy, you will need to arrange for someone to drive you home after the procedure, as the anesthesia used during the procedure can make you drowsy or disoriented.

You should also wear loose, comfortable clothing to the procedure and bring a list of any medications you are taking.

Stay Hydrated

Staying hydrated is essential before and after a colonoscopy. You should drink plenty of clear fluids, such as water, tea, and broth, before the procedure to prevent dehydration.

After the procedure, you may need to drink more fluids than usual to help your body recover from the laxatives or other medications used to clean out your colon.

Follow Post-Procedure Instructions

After the colonoscopy, your doctor will give you specific instructions on how to care for yourself at home. You may need to avoid solid foods for a few hours or take other medications to help manage any discomfort.

It is important to follow your doctor's instructions carefully to ensure that you recover from the procedure as quickly and safely as possible.

Dietary Restrictions

Dietary restrictions are an essential part of preparing for a colonoscopy. The purpose of the restrictions is to clear out your colon, allowing the doctor to examine the lining of the colon for any abnormalities, such as polyps or inflammation. Here are some tips for following the dietary restrictions for a colonoscopy:

Follow Your Doctor's Instructions

Before undergoing a colonoscopy, your doctor will give you specific instructions on how to prepare for the procedure, including any dietary restrictions. It is essential to follow your doctor's instructions carefully to ensure that your colon is adequately cleaned out before the procedure.

Start the Pre-Procedure Diet Early

The pre-procedure diet typically involves avoiding solid foods and drinking clear liquids, such as water, tea, and broth. You may also need to take laxatives or other medications to help clean out your colon.

It is important to start the pre-procedure diet early to ensure that your colon is adequately cleaned out before the procedure. Depending on your doctor's instructions, you may need to follow the pre-procedure diet for one to three days before the colonoscopy.

Avoid Certain Foods and Drinks

During the pre-procedure diet, you will need to avoid certain foods and drinks, such as:

1. Solid foods: You should avoid all solid foods, including fruits, vegetables, and meat.

2. Dairy products: You should avoid all dairy products, including milk, cheese, and yogurt.

3. Fiber: You should avoid all high-fiber foods, such as whole grains, nuts, and seeds.

4. Alcohol: You should avoid all alcoholic beverages.

5. Carbonated beverages: You should avoid all carbonated beverages, such as soda and sparkling water.

Drink Plenty of Clear Liquids

During the pre-procedure diet, you should drink plenty of clear liquids to stay hydrated and prevent dehydration. Clear liquids include:

Water

Tea

Broth

Clear sports drinks

Clear fruit juices (such as apple juice)

You should avoid any liquids with red or purple coloring, as these can resemble blood in the colon and may interfere with the procedure.

Follow Post-Procedure Diet Instructions

After the colonoscopy, your doctor may give you specific instructions on how to transition back to a regular diet. You may need to avoid certain foods or eat a low-fiber diet for a few days after the procedure.

It is important to follow your doctor's instructions carefully to ensure that you recover from the procedure as quickly and safely as possible.

Bowel Preparation Solutions

Bowel preparation is an essential part of preparing for a colonoscopy. The purpose of bowel preparation is to clean out your colon, allowing the doctor to examine the lining of the colon for any abnormalities, such as polyps or inflammation. Bowel preparation solutions are medications that are used to help clean out your colon before a colonoscopy. Here are some things to know about bowel preparation solutions:

Types of Bowel Preparation Solutions

There are several types of bowel preparation solutions available, including:

1. Polyethylene glycol (PEG) solutions: PEG solutions are the most commonly used bowel preparation solutions. They work by drawing water into the colon, causing diarrhea and flushing out the contents of the colon.

2. Sodium phosphate solutions: Sodium phosphate solutions are less commonly used because they can cause electrolyte imbalances and dehydration. They work by drawing water into the colon and increasing bowel movements.

3. Magnesium citrate: Magnesium citrate is a liquid bowel preparation solution that is used in combination with other medications. It works by drawing water into the colon and causing diarrhea.

How to Take Bowel Preparation Solutions

Bowel preparation solutions are typically taken in the evening before the colonoscopy. Your doctor will give you specific instructions on how to take the medication, including the dosage and timing.

Most bowel preparation solutions are mixed with water or another clear liquid and then consumed. Some solutions may need to be chilled before drinking to improve their taste.

It is essential to follow your doctor's instructions carefully and to drink plenty of clear liquids to prevent dehydration.

Side Effects of Bowel Preparation Solutions

Bowel preparation solutions can cause a variety of side effects, including:

Nausea and vomiting

Bloating

Abdominal cramps

Dehydration

Headaches

It is essential to drink plenty of clear liquids and to follow your doctor's instructions carefully to minimize these side effects.

Precautions and Risks

Bowel preparation solutions should be used with caution in people with certain medical conditions, such as kidney disease, heart disease, or electrolyte imbalances.

In rare cases, bowel preparation solutions can cause serious side effects, such as dehydration, electrolyte imbalances, and kidney damage. It is essential to follow your doctor's instructions carefully and to notify them if you experience any unusual symptoms or side effects.

Medication Adjustments

Before undergoing a colonoscopy, it is essential to inform your doctor of any medications you are taking, including over-the-counter medications, supplements, and vitamins. Some medications may need to be adjusted or stopped before the procedure to ensure that the procedure is safe and effective. Here are some things to know about medication adjustments before a colonoscopy:

Types of Medications that may Need to be Adjusted

There are several types of medications that may need to be adjusted before a colonoscopy, including:

1. Blood thinners: Blood thinners, such as warfarin or aspirin, may need to be stopped before the procedure to prevent excessive bleeding during the procedure.

2. Insulin and other diabetes medications: These medications may need to be adjusted to prevent low blood sugar levels during the pre-procedure diet.

3. Nonsteroidal anti-inflammatory drugs (NSAIDs): These medications, including ibuprofen and naproxen, may need to be stopped before the procedure to prevent bleeding during the procedure.

4. Iron supplements: These supplements may need to be stopped before the procedure because they can discolor the colon, making it difficult to detect abnormalities.

Timing of Medication Adjustments

The timing of medication adjustments will depend on the medication and the procedure's timing. Some medications may need to be stopped or adjusted several days before the procedure, while others may need to be stopped only a few days before the procedure.

It is essential to talk to your doctor about any medication adjustments well in advance of the procedure to ensure that there is enough time to adjust your medication regimen.

Importance of Informing Your Doctor

It is essential to inform your doctor of any medications you are taking, including over-the-counter medications, supplements, and vitamins. Some medications can interact with the anesthesia used during the procedure or affect the results of the procedure.

It is important to be honest and upfront with your doctor about any medications you are taking to ensure that the procedure is safe and effective.

Risks of Medication Adjustments

Stopping or adjusting medications before a procedure can pose certain risks, such as:

5. Increased risk of blood clots: Stopping blood thinners can increase the risk of blood clots in some people.

6. Increased risk of infection: Stopping some medications, such as immunosuppressants, can increase the risk of infection.

It is important to talk to your doctor about any potential risks of stopping or adjusting medications before the procedure.

Shared Decision-Making

Shared decision-making (SDM) is a process that involves both the patient and healthcare provider in making informed decisions about treatment options based on the patient's preferences and values. This approach to care has become increasingly important in the field of colonoscopy, as it can help patients make more informed decisions about screening for colorectal cancer.

Colonoscopy is a widely used screening test for colorectal cancer, which is the third most common cancer in both men and women in the United States. Despite its effectiveness, colonoscopy is not without risks, which can include bleeding, perforation, and adverse reactions to anesthesia. As such, it is important for patients to be fully informed of the risks and benefits of the procedure before making a decision about whether or not to undergo it.

The SDM process involves several steps, including identifying the decision that needs to be made, discussing the options, and considering the patient's preferences and values. In the context of colonoscopy, the SDM process may involve a discussion between the patient and healthcare provider about the benefits and risks of the procedure, as well as any alternative screening methods that may be available.

One important aspect of the SDM process is ensuring that the patient fully understands the risks and benefits of the procedure. For example, patients should be informed about the risk of complications such as bleeding and perforation, as well as the potential benefits of detecting and removing precancerous polyps. Patients should also be informed of alternative screening methods, such as fecal occult blood testing or CT colonography, and the relative risks and benefits of these options.

In addition to discussing the risks and benefits of the procedure, the SDM process also involves considering the patient's preferences and values. For example, some patients may be more willing to accept the risks of a colonoscopy in order to obtain the most accurate screening results, while others may be more comfortable with less invasive screening methods, even if they are not as sensitive.

The SDM process may also involve considering the patient's overall health and medical history. For example, elderly patients or those with certain medical conditions may be at higher risk for complications from the procedure, and the risks and benefits may need to be carefully weighed in these cases.

Ultimately, the goal of the SDM process is to ensure that the patient is fully informed and able to make a decision that aligns with their preferences and values. This can help to improve patient satisfaction and reduce the likelihood of regret or dissatisfaction with the decision.

Costs and Insurance Coverage

Costs and insurance coverage are important considerations for anyone who is planning to undergo a colonoscopy. A colonoscopy is a medical procedure that is used to examine the inside of the large intestine (colon) for signs of cancer or other abnormalities. The procedure can be performed in a hospital or outpatient setting, and the cost can vary depending on a number of factors. Below we will discuss the costs and insurance coverage for colonoscopies, as well as strategies to manage these costs.

The cost of a colonoscopy can vary depending on the location of the facility, the type of insurance, and the reason for the procedure. According to Healthcare Bluebook, the fair price for a colonoscopy ranges from $763 to $3,963, with an average cost of $1,764. This price includes the cost of the procedure, anesthesia, and facility fee. However, it does not include the cost of pre-procedure consultations, lab work, or follow-up care.

For patients without insurance, the cost of a colonoscopy can be prohibitively expensive. However, many insurance plans cover the cost of the procedure. Under the Affordable Care Act, all insurance plans are required to cover screening colonoscopies for patients aged 50 and older with no cost-sharing. This means that patients with insurance will not have to pay anything out of pocket for the procedure if it is being done for screening purposes.

Patients who are having a colonoscopy for diagnostic reasons may have to pay a portion of the cost, depending on their insurance plan. Diagnostic colonoscopies are performed when a patient has symptoms such as rectal bleeding, abdominal pain, or a change in bowel habits. Insurance plans may require patients to pay a deductible or coinsurance for diagnostic procedures.

Patients who are uninsured or underinsured may be eligible for financial assistance. Many hospitals and clinics offer financial assistance programs for patients who cannot afford to pay for their medical care. These programs are often based on a patient's income and can provide discounts or free care.

Patients who are concerned about the cost of a colonoscopy can take several steps to manage their expenses. First, they can shop around for the best price. Patients can call different facilities and ask for the cost of the procedure, including the facility fee, anesthesia, and any other fees. Patients can also ask about discounts for self-pay patients or payment plans.

Second, patients can work with their healthcare provider to find alternatives to a colonoscopy. There are several other screening tests for colon cancer that are less expensive than a colonoscopy. These include the fecal immunochemical test (FIT) and the fecal occult blood test (FOBT). However, it is important to note that these tests are less accurate than a colonoscopy and may need to be done more frequently.

Finally, patients can work with their insurance provider to ensure that their colonoscopy is covered by their plan. Patients should contact their insurance provider to verify their coverage and to understand any costs that they may be responsible for. Patients can also ask their provider for a pre-authorization or pre-certification for the procedure to ensure that it is covered by their plan.

Understanding Procedure Costs

Colonoscopy is a medical procedure that allows doctors to examine the lining of the colon and rectum using a flexible, lighted tube with a small camera on the end. This procedure can detect abnormalities such as polyps, ulcers, or tumors that may be cancerous or precancerous. However, like any medical procedure, there are costs involved. Understanding the costs associated with colonoscopy can help patients make informed decisions about their health care.

The cost of a colonoscopy can vary widely depending on several factors, including geographic location, the facility where the procedure is performed, the type of insurance coverage the patient has, and the reason for the procedure. Generally, a routine colonoscopy is less expensive than a diagnostic colonoscopy.

Routine colonoscopies are typically recommended for individuals who are at average risk for developing colon cancer and are over the age of 50. These procedures are considered preventive care and are covered by most insurance plans. However, patients should check with their insurance provider to understand their specific coverage and out-of-pocket costs.

Diagnostic colonoscopies are performed when a patient has symptoms such as rectal bleeding, abdominal pain, or a change in bowel habits. These procedures may also be recommended for individuals with a family history of colon cancer or other risk factors. Diagnostic colonoscopies may be more expensive than routine colonoscopies, as they may require additional testing or procedures.

In addition to the cost of the procedure itself, patients may also incur costs associated with the preparation for the colonoscopy. This may include bowel preparation kits, medications, and other supplies. Patients should check with their insurance provider to understand which of these costs are covered and which may be considered out-of-pocket expenses.

Patients without insurance coverage may face higher costs for colonoscopies. However, many healthcare providers and facilities offer payment plans or financial assistance programs for patients who are unable to pay the full cost of the procedure.

It is important to note that the cost of a colonoscopy should not deter patients from receiving this important screening test. Colon cancer is highly treatable when detected early, and colonoscopies remain the gold standard for detecting and preventing colon cancer. Patients should talk with their healthcare provider about the need for a colonoscopy and work with their insurance provider to understand their coverage and costs.

Insurance Considerations

Insurance Considerations When Getting a Colonoscopy

Colonoscopy is a critical medical procedure that helps detect and prevent colorectal cancer, the second leading cause of cancer-related deaths in the United States. According to the American Cancer Society, people of average risk for colorectal cancer should start getting screened at the age of 45. However, many people avoid getting a colonoscopy due to concerns about the costs associated with the procedure. Below we will discuss insurance considerations when getting a colonoscopy, including insurance coverage and costs.

Insurance Coverage

The Affordable Care Act (ACA) mandates that health insurance plans must cover preventive services, including colonoscopies, without any cost-sharing requirements such as copayments or deductibles. This means that people with private health insurance plans should not have to pay anything out of pocket for a screening colonoscopy, as long as the procedure is considered preventive and meets certain guidelines.

However, the coverage and requirements may vary based on individual insurance plans. Some plans may have different coverage for in-network versus out-of-network providers, and some may require a referral from a primary care physician. Therefore, it is important to contact your insurance provider to verify your specific coverage before scheduling a colonoscopy.

Additionally, Medicare, the federal health insurance program for people over 65, covers screening colonoscopies for eligible beneficiaries. Medicare Part B covers the procedure once every 24 months for people at average risk for colorectal cancer, and once every 12 months for people at high risk. Medicare beneficiaries are responsible for 20% of the Medicare-approved amount for the procedure.

Costs

Despite the insurance coverage requirements for preventive services, some people may still incur costs associated with a colonoscopy. This is because not all colonoscopies are considered preventive, and some diagnostic colonoscopies may be needed if a patient has symptoms or a family history of colorectal cancer.

Diagnostic colonoscopies are considered medically necessary and may be subject to cost-sharing requirements under some insurance plans. The cost-sharing requirements may include a copayment, deductible, or coinsurance, which are the out-of-pocket costs that patients must pay. The amount of cost-sharing varies based on the insurance plan and the individual's deductible and copayment amounts.

In addition to the cost-sharing requirements, patients may also incur costs for pre-procedure consultations, anesthesia, and facility fees. These costs can add up quickly and may vary based on the provider, location, and insurance plan.

However, there are options available for patients who cannot afford the out-of-pocket costs associated with a colonoscopy. For example, some clinics and hospitals offer financial assistance or payment plans for eligible patients. Additionally, some states have programs that offer free or low-cost colonoscopies for uninsured or underinsured individuals.

Financial Assistance Options

Financial Assistance Options for Colonoscopy

Colonoscopy is a vital procedure for the detection and prevention of colon cancer. However, the cost of this procedure may be a significant barrier for some individuals who may not have access to medical insurance or financial resources. Fortunately, there are financial assistance options available for patients who need a colonoscopy. This chapter will explore the different financial assistance options available for colonoscopy and how to access them.

One of the most common ways to get financial assistance for colonoscopy is through health insurance. Most health insurance plans provide coverage for colonoscopies for individuals who meet certain criteria, such as age or risk factors for colon cancer. Patients can check with their insurance providers to understand their coverage and any co-pays or deductibles they may need to pay.

For individuals who do not have health insurance, or whose insurance does not cover colonoscopies, there are other options available. One of the most popular programs is Medicaid, a federal and state-funded program that provides medical coverage for low-income individuals and families. Eligibility criteria vary by state, but generally, individuals with low incomes, disabilities, or other qualifying conditions can receive coverage for colonoscopies through Medicaid.

In addition to Medicaid, there are also several government-funded programs that provide financial assistance for colonoscopies. The National Colorectal Cancer Roundtable (NCCRT) has a program called "80% by 2018" that aims to increase the number of adults aged 50 and older who are up-to-date with recommended colon cancer screening. This program includes funding for low-income individuals to access colonoscopy services. Patients can check with their healthcare providers or local health departments to see if they qualify for this program.

Some healthcare facilities also offer financial assistance programs for colonoscopies. These programs are designed to help individuals who are uninsured, underinsured, or who have financial hardships. These programs can include discounts, payment plans, or even free colonoscopy services. Patients can check with their healthcare provider or the hospital's financial assistance office to learn more about these programs and to apply for financial assistance.

Community-based organizations and non-profit organizations are also good resources for individuals seeking financial assistance for colonoscopies. For example, the American Cancer Society's (ACS) Cancer Resource Network provides a wide range of services, including information about financial resources for cancer patients. Similarly, the Patient Advocate Foundation (PAF) provides free case management services to patients who have chronic, life-threatening, or debilitating illnesses, including colon cancer. Patients can contact these organizations to learn more about financial assistance programs they offer and how to apply.

Finally, patients can also consider clinical trials as a way to access free or low-cost colonoscopies. Clinical trials are research studies that test new treatments or procedures, and they often provide medical services to patients for free or at a reduced cost. Patients can search for clinical trials in their area and see if they meet the eligibility criteria.

Quality Measures in Colonoscopy

Colonoscopy is an essential procedure for the early detection and prevention of colorectal cancer. However, the effectiveness of the colonoscopy depends on the quality of the examination. Quality measures in colonoscopy are essential to ensure that patients receive the highest quality of care possible. Below we will discuss the quality measures in colonoscopy and their importance in improving patient outcomes.

One of the most critical quality measures in colonoscopy is the adenoma detection rate (ADR). The ADR is the percentage of patients who have at least one adenomatous polyp detected during colonoscopy. Adenomas are pre-cancerous growths that, if left untreated, can develop into colorectal cancer. Therefore, the ADR is an essential quality measure for detecting and preventing colorectal cancer. The American Society for Gastrointestinal Endoscopy (ASGE) recommends an ADR of at least 25% for male patients and 15% for female patients. If the ADR falls below these thresholds, it may indicate that the colonoscopy was not thorough enough or that the physician did not have sufficient skill in detecting adenomas.

Another quality measure in colonoscopy is the cecal intubation rate (CIR). The CIR is the percentage of colonoscopies that successfully reach the cecum, the final section of the colon. A high CIR is essential because it ensures that the entire colon is visualized and examined. The ASGE recommends a CIR of at least 90% for screening colonoscopies and 95% for diagnostic colonoscopies. If the CIR falls below these thresholds, it may indicate that the colonoscopy was incomplete or that the physician lacked the necessary skill or experience to reach the cecum.

Another important quality measure in colonoscopy is the withdrawal time. The withdrawal time is the amount of time the physician takes to examine the colon during the withdrawal of the colonoscope. A longer withdrawal time is associated with higher ADR and improved detection of adenomas. The ASGE recommends a withdrawal time of at least six minutes. A shorter withdrawal time may indicate that the physician did not take enough time to carefully examine the colon or that the colonoscopy was rushed.

The bowel preparation is also an essential factor in the quality of a colonoscopy. Adequate bowel preparation is necessary to ensure that the colon is clean and that the physician can see the colon's lining clearly. Inadequate bowel preparation can result in missed adenomas or an incomplete examination of the colon. The ASGE recommends that patients receive a high-quality bowel preparation that ensures adequate cleansing of the colon. Patients should follow the bowel preparation instructions carefully and notify their physician if they have any difficulties with the preparation.

Another quality measure in colonoscopy is the use of sedation. Sedation can improve patient comfort during the procedure, but excessive sedation can result in complications such as respiratory depression or cardiac events. The ASGE recommends that sedation is administered by a trained healthcare provider who can monitor the patient's vital signs and ensure that the sedation is appropriate for the patient's medical condition.

In addition to the above quality measures, there are several other factors that can impact the quality of a colonoscopy. These include the use of high-definition imaging technology, the experience and skill of the physician, and the use of appropriate follow-up procedures after the colonoscopy. Patients should choose a qualified physician who has a high ADR and CIR and who uses high-definition imaging technology to visualize the colon's lining.

Adenoma Detection Rate

Adenomas are a type of polyp that can develop in the colon or rectum, and they have the potential to become cancerous if left untreated. Adenoma detection rate (ADR) is a measure of how effectively colonoscopies detect these precancerous polyps. This metric is widely regarded as a key quality measure for colonoscopy, as the detection and removal of adenomas can significantly reduce the risk of developing colorectal cancer.

The ADR is calculated by dividing the number of patients with at least one adenoma detected during a colonoscopy by the total number of patients who underwent the procedure. A high ADR is generally considered desirable, as it indicates that the colonoscopist is thorough in their examination and is more likely to detect and remove adenomas. The American Society for Gastrointestinal Endoscopy (ASGE) recommends a minimum ADR of 25% for male patients and 15% for female patients.

Several factors can influence ADR, including patient age, sex, and overall health, as well as the quality of the colonoscopy and the experience and skill of the colonoscopist. Studies have shown that ADR tends to be higher in older patients, particularly those over the age of 60, and in male patients compared to female patients. A history of polyps or colorectal cancer in the patient or their family can also increase the likelihood of adenomas being detected during colonoscopy.

To improve ADR, colonoscopists must carefully examine the colon and rectum, using a variety of techniques to detect adenomas. These techniques include careful inspection of the mucosa, withdrawal of the scope at a slow and steady pace, and use of specialized tools such as chromoendoscopy, which involves staining the tissue to enhance visualization of abnormalities. It is also important to carefully document the findings of the colonoscopy, as this can help identify areas where improvement is needed.

The importance of ADR as a quality measure for colonoscopy cannot be overstated. Studies have consistently shown that a higher ADR is associated with a lower risk of colorectal cancer. One study found that patients whose colonoscopists had an ADR of less than 15% were more than twice as likely to develop colorectal cancer within five years of the procedure compared to patients whose colonoscopists had an ADR of 25% or higher. Another study found that a 1% increase in ADR was associated with a 3% reduction in the risk of developing colorectal cancer.

Given the importance of ADR, there has been a growing emphasis on measuring and reporting this metric as part of efforts to improve the quality of colonoscopy. Several organizations, including the ASGE and the American College of Gastroenterology (ACG), have developed programs to promote high-quality colonoscopy and to help colonoscopists improve their ADR. These programs often involve ongoing monitoring and feedback on ADR, as well as education and training on techniques to improve adenoma detection.

In addition to ADR, other quality measures for colonoscopy include cecal intubation rate (CIR), which measures how often the colonoscope is advanced to the cecum, the furthest point in the colon, and withdrawal time, which measures the time it takes to withdraw the colonoscope from the colon. These measures can also impact the overall effectiveness of colonoscopy in detecting and preventing colorectal cancer.

Cecal Intubation Rate

Cecal intubation is a critical aspect of colonoscopy, as it determines whether the entire colon has been visualized and any abnormalities have been detected. Below we will explore the importance of cecal intubation rate in colonoscopy, the factors that affect it, and strategies to improve it.

Cecal intubation is the process of advancing the colonoscope through the colon to the cecum, which is the first part of the large intestine. The cecum is where the small intestine connects to the large intestine, and the ileocecal valve separates the two. Cecal intubation is important in colonoscopy because it enables the visualization of the entire colon, including the ascending colon, transverse colon, descending colon, and sigmoid colon.

The cecal intubation rate (CIR) is defined as the percentage of colonoscopies in which the colonoscope reaches the cecum. The American Society for Gastrointestinal Endoscopy (ASGE) recommends a minimum CIR of 90% for screening colonoscopies and 95% for diagnostic colonoscopies. Achieving a high CIR is crucial for the accuracy and effectiveness of colonoscopy in detecting and preventing colorectal cancer.

Several factors can affect the CIR in colonoscopy. Patient factors such as a history of prior abdominal surgery, obesity, and poor bowel preparation can make it challenging to reach the cecum. Operator factors such as lack of experience, poor technique, and inadequate sedation can also affect the CIR. In addition, anatomical factors such as tortuosity or redundancy of the colon can make it difficult to advance the colonoscope to the cecum.

To improve the CIR in colonoscopy, several strategies can be implemented. First, adequate bowel preparation is essential to optimize the CIR. Patients should be instructed to follow the bowel preparation regimen carefully, and the quality of the preparation should be assessed before the procedure. Second, operators should ensure they have adequate training and experience in colonoscopy, including techniques for maneuvering through the colon. Third, the use of carbon dioxide insufflation during colonoscopy can reduce discomfort and increase patient tolerance, allowing for a more complete examination. Fourth, altering the patient's position, such as placing them in the left lateral decubitus position, can facilitate the advancement of the colonoscope through the colon. Fifth, using an advanced imaging technique, such as narrow-band imaging or chromoendoscopy, can enhance visualization and facilitate the identification of the cecum.

A low CIR can have significant consequences for patients, including missed lesions and the need for repeat procedures. Therefore, it is essential to monitor and improve the CIR in colonoscopy. Quality measures such as the CIR and adenoma detection rate (ADR) are being increasingly used as indicators of colonoscopy quality and effectiveness. Adenoma detection rate refers to the percentage of screening colonoscopies in which at least one adenoma is detected. A high ADR is associated with a lower risk of interval colorectal cancer, which is colorectal cancer that develops between screening colonoscopies.

Withdrawal Time

Withdrawal time refers to the length of time a physician takes to inspect the entire colon during a colonoscopy. This is a critical measure of the quality of the procedure, as it affects the ability to detect and remove polyps, and ultimately, prevent colorectal cancer. Below we will explore what withdrawal time is, why it is important, how it is measured, and how it can be improved.

During a colonoscopy, a flexible tube with a light and camera, called a colonoscope, is inserted through the rectum and navigated through the colon to look for polyps or other abnormalities. The physician will carefully inspect the colon during insertion and removal of the colonoscope. The withdrawal time refers to the time the physician spends examining the colon during the removal phase of the colonoscopy.

The importance of withdrawal time lies in the ability to detect and remove precancerous polyps. Studies have shown that longer withdrawal times are associated with higher rates of adenoma detection, or the ability to detect precancerous polyps. Additionally, research has demonstrated that a shorter withdrawal time is associated with an increased risk of missed polyps, which could lead to a delayed diagnosis of colorectal cancer.

To ensure quality colonoscopies, gastroenterology societies recommend a minimum withdrawal time of 6 minutes. This time allows for a thorough inspection of the colon and increases the likelihood of detecting and removing polyps. However, some studies have suggested that a withdrawal time of at least 8 minutes may be even more effective.

Withdrawal time is measured by the colonoscopy technician, who uses a timer to record the length of time the physician spends inspecting the colon during the removal phase of the procedure. The measurement starts when the colonoscope is fully inserted into the cecum, which is the beginning of the colon. The timer is stopped when the colonoscope is removed from the anus.

To improve withdrawal time, there are several strategies that can be implemented. One approach is to ensure that the physician performing the colonoscopy is experienced and trained in detecting polyps. Additionally, using high-definition colonoscopes and narrow band imaging can increase the ability to detect polyps and potentially decrease the time needed for inspection.

Another strategy is to implement feedback and quality improvement programs to monitor and improve withdrawal time. Feedback can include regular audits and peer review of colonoscopy videos to provide constructive criticism to the physicians performing the procedure. Quality improvement programs can provide education and training to improve technique and ensure that minimum withdrawal time standards are met.

Choosing a Colonoscopy Provider

Choosing a Colonoscopy Provider

Colonoscopy is an essential screening procedure that can help detect and prevent colorectal cancer. Choosing the right colonoscopy provider is crucial to ensure that the procedure is performed safely, accurately, and with the least discomfort. With so many providers available, it can be overwhelming to determine which one to choose. This chapter aims to provide an informative guide to help patients choose the right colonoscopy provider.

Accreditation and Certification

When looking for a colonoscopy provider, the first thing to check is their accreditation and certification. Accreditation ensures that the provider meets the standards set by regulatory bodies such as the Joint Commission or the Accreditation Association for Ambulatory Health Care (AAAHC). Certification indicates that the provider has undergone specific training and has met the requirements set by the American Society for Gastrointestinal Endoscopy (ASGE) or the American College of Gastroenterology (ACG). These credentials are essential as they ensure that the provider has the necessary skills, expertise, and equipment to perform the procedure safely and effectively.

Experience and Expertise

Another crucial factor to consider when choosing a colonoscopy provider is their experience and expertise. It is important to choose a provider who has performed a significant number of colonoscopies and has the necessary training and expertise in detecting and removing polyps. A provider who is well-versed in the latest techniques and technologies and is up-to-date with current guidelines is more likely to provide an accurate diagnosis and ensure that the patient receives the best possible care.

Quality of Care

The quality of care provided by a colonoscopy provider is another important consideration. Patients should look for providers who offer personalized care and are committed to providing the highest level of service. It is important to choose a provider who takes the time to explain the procedure, answers all questions and concerns, and ensures that the patient feels comfortable throughout the process. The provider should also provide clear instructions on pre-procedure preparation, post-procedure care, and follow-up appointments.

Facility and Equipment

The facility and equipment used by a colonoscopy provider are crucial to ensuring the safety and success of the procedure. Patients should look for providers who operate in state-of-the-art facilities that are clean, well-maintained, and have modern equipment. The facility should also have an experienced and trained staff that is equipped to handle emergencies and complications that may arise during the procedure.

Cost and Insurance Coverage

Cost and insurance coverage are also essential considerations when choosing a colonoscopy provider. Patients should compare prices and ensure that the provider they choose offers competitive rates without compromising on quality. It is also important to check with their insurance company to ensure that the procedure is covered and to understand their out-of-pocket expenses.

Patient Reviews and Recommendations

Finally, patient reviews and recommendations can provide valuable insights into the quality of care provided by a colonoscopy provider. Patients can check online reviews on websites such as Yelp or Google, or ask for recommendations from friends, family, or their primary care physician. These reviews can provide valuable feedback on the provider's bedside manner, quality of care, and overall patient experience.

Credentials and Experience

Colonoscopy is a vital tool in the early detection and prevention of colon cancer. It is important to ensure that the colonoscopy is performed by a qualified and experienced healthcare professional. Patients should be aware of the credentials and experience of the healthcare professional who will be performing the colonoscopy to make informed decisions.

The healthcare professional who performs the colonoscopy should be a gastroenterologist, a medical doctor who specializes in the diagnosis and treatment of digestive disorders. They must have completed a medical degree and residency in internal medicine, followed by a fellowship in gastroenterology. This fellowship involves three years of intensive training in the diagnosis and treatment of gastrointestinal diseases, including colonoscopy. Gastroenterologists are also required to be board-certified by the American Board of Internal Medicine.

In addition to a gastroenterologist, a surgeon may also perform colonoscopy, particularly if the patient has a history of colon cancer or other gastrointestinal conditions that require surgery. Surgeons who perform colonoscopy must also have specialized training and certification in the procedure.

It is also important to consider the experience of the healthcare professional performing the colonoscopy. Studies have shown that the adenoma detection rate, or the percentage of patients who have adenomas (precancerous polyps) detected during a colonoscopy, is higher in healthcare professionals who perform a high volume of colonoscopies per year. Therefore, patients may wish to consider healthcare professionals who perform a high volume of colonoscopies.

Patients should also consider the reputation of the healthcare professional and the facility where the colonoscopy will be performed. It is important to choose a reputable facility with a strong track record of success in performing colonoscopies.

Before undergoing a colonoscopy, patients should feel comfortable asking their healthcare professional questions about their credentials and experience. They may also wish to research the healthcare professional online and read reviews from other patients.

In addition to the healthcare professional who performs the colonoscopy, it is also important to consider the team that will be supporting the procedure. The team should include trained nurses and technicians who are experienced in assisting with colonoscopies and monitoring patients during the procedure.

Facility Accreditation

Facility accreditation is a critical aspect to consider when choosing a facility for a colonoscopy procedure. Accreditation is a process by which a healthcare facility is assessed by an independent organization to determine whether it meets certain predetermined standards. In the case of colonoscopy facilities, accreditation is typically carried out by the Accreditation Association for Ambulatory Health Care (AAAHC) or the Joint Commission.

Accreditation is important because it ensures that the facility provides a high level of care and adheres to strict safety standards. It also demonstrates a commitment to continuous quality improvement and patient-centered care. Accredited facilities are subject to regular inspections to ensure that they continue to meet these standards.

One of the primary benefits of choosing an accredited facility for a colonoscopy procedure is the assurance that the facility has the necessary equipment and resources to perform the procedure safely and effectively. Accredited facilities are required to have state-of-the-art equipment and to follow strict guidelines for infection prevention and control. This can help to reduce the risk of complications and ensure that the procedure is conducted in a safe and effective manner.

Another benefit of choosing an accredited facility is the quality of the staff. Accredited facilities are required to have highly trained and qualified staff who are knowledgeable about the latest developments in colonoscopy procedures and techniques. This can help to ensure that patients receive the highest level of care possible and that any complications or issues that arise during the procedure are handled quickly and effectively.

Accredited facilities are also required to have policies and procedures in place to protect patient privacy and confidentiality. This is important because colonoscopy procedures are sensitive and involve the use of personal and sensitive information. Accredited facilities are required to follow strict guidelines for the collection, use, and storage of patient information to ensure that it remains confidential and is not shared without the patient's consent.

When choosing a facility for a colonoscopy procedure, it is important to look for one that is accredited by a recognized organization such as the AAAHC or the Joint Commission. Accreditation provides assurance that the facility has met rigorous standards for quality and safety and that it is committed to providing the highest level of care possible. Patients should also look for a facility with a well-trained and experienced staff, state-of-the-art equipment, and policies and procedures in place to protect patient privacy and confidentiality.

It is also important to consider other factors such as the location of the facility, its hours of operation, and the availability of appointments. Patients should choose a facility that is convenient to their home or workplace and that offers flexible scheduling options to accommodate their needs.

In summary, facility accreditation is a critical factor to consider when choosing a facility for a colonoscopy procedure. Accreditation provides assurance that the facility has met rigorous standards for quality and safety and is committed to providing the highest level of care possible. Patients should look for an accredited facility with a well-trained and experienced staff, state-of-the-art equipment, and policies and procedures in place to protect patient privacy and confidentiality.

Patient Satisfaction

Colonoscopy is a medical procedure that is used to examine the colon and rectum for abnormalities or signs of diseases such as colon cancer. While the procedure itself is important, the patient experience and satisfaction with the procedure are also crucial. Below we will explore the importance of patient satisfaction during a colonoscopy and how it can impact the overall success of the procedure.

Patient satisfaction during a colonoscopy can have a significant impact on the success of the procedure. Patients who are satisfied with their experience are more likely to adhere to the recommended follow-up screenings and continue to seek regular medical care. In contrast, patients who are dissatisfied may be less likely to adhere to the recommended screening and follow-up care, which can lead to missed diagnoses and poor health outcomes.

There are several factors that can impact patient satisfaction during a colonoscopy. One important factor is communication between the patient and healthcare provider. Patients who feel that their healthcare provider is listening to them, taking their concerns seriously, and providing clear and detailed information about the procedure are more likely to feel satisfied with their experience.

Another important factor is patient comfort during the procedure. Patients who experience minimal discomfort during the colonoscopy are more likely to feel satisfied with their experience. This can be achieved through the use of appropriate sedation and pain management techniques, as well as ensuring that the patient is positioned comfortably during the procedure.

Facility environment and cleanliness can also impact patient satisfaction. Patients who feel that the facility is clean, organized, and well-maintained are more likely to feel satisfied with their experience. Additionally, a welcoming and calming environment can help to reduce patient anxiety and improve their overall experience.

It is important to note that patient satisfaction during a colonoscopy is not just important for the patient, but also for the healthcare provider and facility. Satisfied patients are more likely to recommend the facility and healthcare provider to others, which can lead to increased referrals and revenue. In contrast, dissatisfied patients may share their negative experience with others, leading to a loss of potential patients and revenue.

To ensure patient satisfaction during a colonoscopy, healthcare providers and facilities can take several steps. First, communication with the patient should be a top priority. This includes providing clear and detailed information about the procedure, as well as answering any questions or concerns that the patient may have. Additionally, healthcare providers should ensure that the patient is comfortable throughout the procedure, using appropriate sedation and pain management techniques.

The facility environment should also be clean, organized, and welcoming. This can be achieved through regular maintenance and cleaning, as well as the use of calming decor and comfortable furnishings. Additionally, healthcare providers should take steps to ensure that the patient feels respected and valued, such as addressing them by their preferred name and avoiding rushing through the procedure.

What can I expect after my colonoscopy?

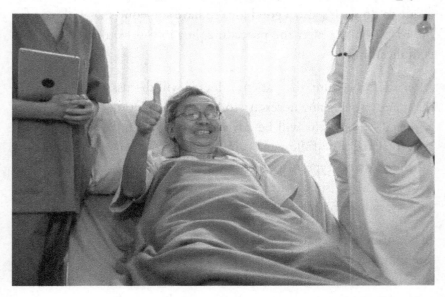

After a colonoscopy, patients can expect to experience some mild discomfort and side effects, but these typically resolve quickly. The recovery process is generally short, and most people can resume their normal activities the next day. However, it's important to follow the instructions given by your doctor, as every case and person is different.

Immediately after the procedure, patients will be taken to a recovery area where they will be monitored until the sedation wears off. During this time, patients may experience mild cramping or bloating as a result of the air that was used to inflate the colon during the procedure. This discomfort should resolve quickly, and patients will be able to eat and drink as soon as they feel ready.

It's important to note that patients should not drive or operate heavy machinery for the rest of the day, or until their doctor advises them it is safe to do so. It's also a good idea to have someone stay with you for the first 24 hours after the procedure, just in case you experience any complications.

After the procedure, the patient's doctor will discuss the results with them and provide any necessary follow-up instructions. If polyps were removed, the patient will be advised to have them tested for cancer and to schedule a follow-up colonoscopy in a few years, depending on the size and type of polyp. If cancer was found, the patient will be referred to a specialist for further treatment, which may include surgery, radiation therapy, and/or chemotherapy.

It is normal to experience mild discomfort such as gas, bloating or cramping for a few hours after the procedure. You may feel a bit tired as well, but these symptoms should resolve within a day or two. You can take over-the-counter pain medication to help with any discomfort. You may also have a mild rectal bleeding or blood in the stool for a day or two after the procedure. It is important to notify your doctor if you have more than a small amount of bleeding, severe abdominal pain, fever, or other symptoms that are concerning.

Most people are able to return to their normal activities the next day, but it's important to avoid strenuous activities, such as heavy lifting, for a day or two after the procedure. It's also important to avoid any foods or drinks that can cause gas or discomfort, such as beans, broccoli, cabbage, and certain fruits, for a day or two after the procedure.

It is also important to follow any other instructions given by your doctor, such as what medications to take or avoid, and what to wear during the procedure. Your doctor may also advise you to avoid alcohol for a day or two after the procedure.

Post-Colonoscopy Care

After a colonoscopy procedure, it is important to take care of oneself in the post-procedure period to ensure a speedy and comfortable recovery. This includes following specific instructions from the healthcare provider, maintaining a healthy diet, and monitoring any potential complications.

Instructions from Healthcare Provider

After the procedure, the healthcare provider will give specific instructions for post-procedure care. This may include:

1. Diet restrictions: The patient may be instructed to avoid certain foods or liquids for a period of time after the procedure. This may include solid foods or certain types of liquids.

2. Medication instructions: The healthcare provider may instruct the patient to temporarily stop taking certain medications or to adjust the dosage.

3. Activity restrictions: The patient may be instructed to avoid strenuous activity or heavy lifting for a period of time after the procedure.

4. Follow-up appointment: The healthcare provider may schedule a follow-up appointment to discuss the results of the procedure and any necessary next steps.

Following these instructions is important to ensure a smooth recovery and avoid any potential complications.

Maintaining a Healthy Diet

Following a colonoscopy, it is important to maintain a healthy diet to promote healing and avoid any potential complications. This may include:

5. Drinking plenty of fluids: The patient should drink plenty of fluids to stay hydrated and help flush out any remaining bowel preparation solution.

6. Eating light, easy-to-digest foods: The patient may want to eat light, easy-to-digest foods such as soups, broths, or cooked vegetables for the first few days after the procedure.

7. Avoiding high-fiber foods: The patient may need to avoid high-fiber foods such as whole grains, fruits, and vegetables for a period of time after the procedure to allow the colon to heal.

8. Gradually resuming normal diet: Once the healthcare provider gives the green light, the patient can gradually resume their normal diet.

Monitoring for Complications

After a colonoscopy, it is important to monitor for any potential complications. This may include:

9. Rectal bleeding: It is normal to experience some mild rectal bleeding after a colonoscopy. However, if the bleeding is excessive or persists for several days, the patient should contact their healthcare provider.

10. Abdominal pain: The patient may experience some mild abdominal pain or discomfort after the procedure. However, if the pain is severe or persistent, the patient should contact their healthcare provider.

11. Fever: A low-grade fever is common after a colonoscopy. However, if the fever is high or persistent, the patient should contact their healthcare provider.

12. Changes in bowel movements: It is normal to experience some changes in bowel movements after a colonoscopy, such as diarrhea or constipation. However, if the changes are severe or persistent, the patient should contact their healthcare provider.

Recovery Process

Recovering from a colonoscopy can vary from person to person, but there are several key factors that can help promote a comfortable and successful recovery. These include taking it easy for the first few days, staying hydrated, and gradually resuming normal activities.

Taking it Easy

After a colonoscopy, it is important to take it easy for the first few days to allow the body to recover. This may include:

1. Resting: The patient should take it easy and rest as much as possible for the first few days after the procedure.

2. Avoiding strenuous activity: The patient should avoid any strenuous activity or heavy lifting for at least a few days after the procedure.

3. Taking time off work: Depending on the nature of the patient's job, they may need to take some time off work to allow their body to recover.

Staying Hydrated

Staying hydrated is important after a colonoscopy to promote healing and prevent dehydration. This may include:

4. Drinking plenty of fluids: The patient should drink plenty of fluids, including water, clear broths, and electrolyte drinks.

5. Avoiding alcohol and caffeine: The patient should avoid alcohol and caffeine for the first few days after the procedure, as these can dehydrate the body.

6. Eating foods with high water content: The patient can also eat foods with high water content, such as fruits and vegetables, to help stay hydrated.

Gradually Resuming Normal Activities

Gradually resuming normal activities can help the patient recover from a colonoscopy and avoid any potential complications. This may include:

7. Starting with light activities: The patient should start with light activities, such as walking, and gradually increase the intensity and duration over time.

8. Resuming normal diet: Once the healthcare provider gives the green light, the patient can gradually resume their normal diet.

9. Following medication instructions: The patient should follow any medication instructions provided by their healthcare provider.

10. Attending follow-up appointments: The patient should attend any follow-up appointments scheduled by their healthcare provider to discuss the results of the procedure and any necessary next steps.

Potential Complications

While colonoscopies are generally safe, there are some potential complications that can occur. These may include:

11. Bleeding: Mild rectal bleeding is common after a colonoscopy, but excessive bleeding may occur in rare cases.

12. Perforation: In rare cases, the colon may become perforated during a colonoscopy, which may require surgical repair.

13. Infection: There is a small risk of infection after a colonoscopy, which can usually be treated with antibiotics.

It is important for patients to contact their healthcare provider if they experience any severe or persistent symptoms after a colonoscopy, such as severe abdominal pain, fever, or bleeding.

Resuming Normal Activities

Resuming normal activities after a colonoscopy is an important part of the recovery process. While it is important to take it easy for the first few days after the procedure, gradually resuming normal activities can help the patient get back to their daily routine and avoid potential complications.

Starting with Light Activities

It is recommended that patients start with light activities after a colonoscopy and gradually increase the intensity and duration over time. This may include:

1. Walking: Walking is a low-impact activity that can help promote healing and prevent blood clots. The patient can start with short walks around the house or neighborhood and gradually increase the distance over time.

2. Stretching: Gentle stretching can help prevent muscle soreness and stiffness after the procedure. The patient can start with simple stretches and gradually increase the intensity over time.

3. Yoga or Pilates: Gentle yoga or Pilates can also help promote flexibility and strength after a colonoscopy. It is important to consult with the healthcare provider before starting any new exercise program.

Resuming Normal Diet

The patient may be instructed to follow a clear liquid diet for the first 24 hours after the colonoscopy to allow the bowel to rest. After this, they can gradually resume their normal diet. It is important to:

4. Start with light, easy-to-digest foods: The patient should start with light, easy-to-digest foods, such as soup, crackers, and toast, and gradually add more solid foods over time.

5. Avoid spicy, greasy, or heavy foods: The patient should avoid spicy, greasy, or heavy foods for the first few days after the procedure to prevent digestive upset.

6. Stay hydrated: It is important to stay hydrated after a colonoscopy by drinking plenty of fluids, such as water, clear broths, and electrolyte drinks.

Following Medication Instructions

The patient should follow any medication instructions provided by their healthcare provider after the colonoscopy. This may include:

7. Taking pain medication as needed: The patient may be prescribed pain medication to manage any discomfort or cramping after the procedure.

8. Continuing any pre-existing medication: The patient should continue taking any pre-existing medication unless instructed otherwise by their healthcare provider.

9. Avoiding blood thinners: The patient should avoid blood thinners, such as aspirin or ibuprofen, for at least a few days after the procedure to prevent bleeding.

Attending Follow-up Appointments

The patient should attend any follow-up appointments scheduled by their healthcare provider after the colonoscopy. This may include:

10. Discussing the results of the procedure: The healthcare provider will discuss the results of the procedure with the patient and any necessary next steps, such as further testing or treatment.

11. Addressing any concerns or questions: The patient can ask any questions or address any concerns they may have about the procedure or their recovery.

Potential Complications

While colonoscopies are generally safe, there are some potential complications that can occur. These may include:

12. Bleeding: Mild rectal bleeding is common after a colonoscopy, but excessive bleeding may occur in rare cases.

13. Perforation: In rare cases, the colon may become perforated during a colonoscopy, which may require surgical repair.

14. Infection: There is a small risk of infection after a colonoscopy, which can usually be treated with antibiotics.

It is important for patients to contact their healthcare provider if they experience any severe or persistent symptoms after a colonoscopy, such as severe abdominal pain, fever, or bleeding.

Managing Discomfort

Colonoscopy is a diagnostic procedure used to examine the colon and rectum for abnormalities, including polyps and signs of colorectal cancer. While the procedure is generally safe, it can cause some discomfort during and after the procedure. Fortunately, there are several ways to manage discomfort during and after a colonoscopy.

During the Procedure

During the procedure, patients may experience some discomfort, such as cramping or bloating, as a result of the air that is used to inflate the colon. This can cause some pressure and discomfort, but there are several ways to manage this discomfort:

1. Breathing Exercises: Deep breathing exercises can help patients relax and reduce feelings of discomfort. Taking slow, deep breaths through the nose and exhaling slowly through the mouth can help ease tension in the body.

2. Relaxation Techniques: Patients can use relaxation techniques such as visualization, progressive muscle relaxation, or guided meditation to help manage discomfort during the procedure.

3. Communication with the Healthcare Provider: Patients should communicate with their healthcare provider about any discomfort they may be experiencing. The healthcare provider may be able to adjust the procedure or provide medication to help manage discomfort.

After the Procedure

After the colonoscopy, patients may experience some discomfort, such as cramping, bloating, or gas. There are several ways to manage this discomfort:

4. Rest: Resting for a few hours after the procedure can help reduce discomfort and promote healing.

5. Pain Medication: Over-the-counter pain medication such as acetaminophen or ibuprofen can help manage discomfort after the procedure. Patients should consult with their healthcare provider before taking any medication.

6. Heating Pad: A heating pad can help reduce discomfort caused by cramping or bloating. Patients should use a low heat setting and avoid placing the heating pad directly on the skin.

7. Hydration: Staying hydrated can help prevent constipation and reduce discomfort. Patients should drink plenty of fluids, such as water or clear broths.

8. Light Diet: Patients should start with a light diet of easily digestible foods, such as soup or crackers, and gradually add more solid foods over time.

It is important for patients to contact their healthcare provider if they experience severe or persistent discomfort after a colonoscopy, such as severe abdominal pain, fever, or bleeding.

Complications

While colonoscopies are generally safe, there are some potential complications that can occur. These may include:

9. Bleeding: Mild rectal bleeding is common after a colonoscopy, but excessive bleeding may occur in rare cases.

10. Perforation: In rare cases, the colon may become perforated during a colonoscopy, which may require surgical repair.

11. Infection: There is a small risk of infection after a colonoscopy, which can usually be treated with antibiotics.

Patients should contact their healthcare provider immediately if they experience any severe or persistent symptoms after a colonoscopy, such as severe abdominal pain, fever, or bleeding.

Understanding Colonoscopy Results

Colonoscopy is a diagnostic procedure that is used to detect abnormalities in the colon and rectum, such as polyps, ulcers, or tumors. During the procedure, a flexible tube with a camera at the end is inserted into the rectum and advanced through the colon. The camera transmits images of the colon and rectum to a monitor, allowing the healthcare provider to examine the lining of the colon for abnormalities. After the procedure, the results of the colonoscopy are typically discussed with the patient. Understanding colonoscopy results is important for patients to be able to make informed decisions about their health.

Normal Colonoscopy Results

A normal colonoscopy result means that no abnormalities were found in the colon or rectum. This is good news and indicates that the patient does not have any serious conditions that need to be addressed. Patients with normal colonoscopy results are typically advised to have another colonoscopy in 10 years, assuming they have no increased risk factors for colorectal cancer.

Abnormal Colonoscopy Results

If abnormalities are found during a colonoscopy, the healthcare provider may take biopsies or remove polyps for further testing. Abnormal results may indicate the presence of a range of conditions, including:

1. Polyps: Polyps are small growths that can be precursors to colorectal cancer. They are typically removed during the colonoscopy and sent for further testing to determine if they are benign or cancerous.

2. Ulcers: Ulcers are sores that can develop in the lining of the colon or rectum. They may be caused by inflammation, infection, or other conditions.

3. Tumors: Tumors are abnormal growths that can be benign or cancerous. If a tumor is detected during a colonoscopy, further testing will be needed to determine if it is cancerous.

4. Inflammatory bowel disease (IBD): IBD is a chronic condition that causes inflammation in the digestive tract. Colonoscopy can help diagnose and monitor IBD.

5. Diverticulosis: Diverticulosis is a condition that causes small pouches to form in the lining of the colon. In some cases, these pouches can become infected or inflamed.

6. Other conditions: Other conditions that may be detected during a colonoscopy include hemorrhoids, fissures, and strictures.

Follow-Up Testing

If abnormal results are found during a colonoscopy, follow-up testing may be needed. This may include additional imaging tests, such as a CT scan or MRI, or blood tests to check for markers of cancer. If polyps are removed during the colonoscopy, the healthcare provider will typically recommend a follow-up colonoscopy in 3-5 years to ensure that no new polyps have formed.

It is important for patients to discuss their results with their healthcare provider to understand the significance of any abnormalities and the recommended follow-up testing. Patients with abnormal results may be referred to a specialist, such as a gastroenterologist or oncologist, for further evaluation and treatment.

Normal Results

A colonoscopy is a diagnostic procedure used to detect abnormalities in the colon and rectum, such as polyps, ulcers, or tumors. During the procedure, a flexible tube with a camera at the end is inserted into the rectum and advanced through the colon. The camera transmits images of the colon and rectum to a monitor, allowing the healthcare provider to examine the lining of the colon for abnormalities. After the procedure, the results of the colonoscopy are typically discussed with the patient. Understanding normal colonoscopy results is important for patients to be able to make informed decisions about their health.

Normal colonoscopy results mean that no abnormalities were found in the colon or rectum. This is good news and indicates that the patient does not have any serious conditions that need to be addressed. It is important to note that while a normal colonoscopy is reassuring, it does not provide a guarantee against developing colorectal cancer in the future. However, regular screening with colonoscopy can help detect and prevent colorectal cancer at an early stage.

The recommended age to begin screening for colorectal cancer with a colonoscopy is 50 for individuals of average risk. Patients with a family history of colorectal cancer or certain genetic conditions may need to begin screening at an earlier age or have more frequent screenings. Patients should discuss their individual risk factors with their healthcare provider to determine the appropriate screening schedule for them.

If a patient has a normal colonoscopy result, they are typically advised to have another colonoscopy in 10 years, assuming they have no increased risk factors for colorectal cancer. However, if the patient has a history of colon cancer or polyps, their healthcare provider may recommend more frequent screenings.

Patients with normal colonoscopy results should continue to maintain a healthy lifestyle to reduce their risk of developing colorectal cancer. This includes eating a diet rich in fruits, vegetables, and whole grains, exercising regularly, not smoking, and limiting alcohol intake.

It is important for patients to follow their healthcare provider's recommendations for screening and maintain open communication with their healthcare provider about any concerns or changes in their health. Regular screening with colonoscopy can help detect and prevent colorectal cancer at an early stage, when it is most treatable.

Abnormal Findings

A colonoscopy is a procedure that is used to examine the lining of the colon and rectum to identify any abnormalities, such as polyps, ulcers, or tumors. Abnormal findings during a colonoscopy can be concerning and may require further testing or treatment. Understanding what abnormal findings can be identified during a colonoscopy is important for patients to be able to make informed decisions about their health.

Some of the abnormal findings that can be identified during a colonoscopy include:

1. Polyps: Polyps are growths that can develop in the lining of the colon or rectum. While most polyps are noncancerous, some may become cancerous over time. During a colonoscopy, polyps can be identified and removed to prevent the development of colon cancer.

2. Ulcers: Ulcers are sores that can develop in the lining of the colon or rectum. They can be caused by inflammation or infection and can be treated with medication.

3. Tumors: Tumors are abnormal growths of cells that can develop in the colon or rectum. They can be either benign (noncancerous) or malignant (cancerous). If a tumor is identified during a colonoscopy, a biopsy may be taken to determine if it is cancerous.

4. Diverticula: Diverticula are small pouches that can develop in the lining of the colon. While they are typically harmless, they can become inflamed or infected, leading to a condition called diverticulitis.

5. Inflammation: Inflammation of the colon, such as in the case of inflammatory bowel disease (IBD), can be identified during a colonoscopy. Treatment for inflammation may involve medication and lifestyle changes.

6. Strictures: Strictures are narrowings of the colon that can cause bowel obstruction. They can be caused by scar tissue from previous surgeries or inflammation.

If abnormal findings are identified during a colonoscopy, additional testing or treatment may be necessary. For example, if polyps are identified, they can be removed during the colonoscopy or a follow-up colonoscopy may be recommended to ensure that no new polyps have developed.

If a biopsy is taken during the colonoscopy, the results may take several days to be processed. Patients should follow up with their healthcare provider to discuss the results and determine any necessary treatment or further testing.

It is important for patients to follow their healthcare provider's recommendations for screening and maintain open communication about any concerns or changes in their health. Regular screening with colonoscopy can help detect and prevent colorectal cancer at an early stage, when it is most treatable.

Recommended Follow-up

Colonoscopy is a valuable diagnostic tool in the detection and prevention of colon and rectal cancer. After the procedure, the doctor will provide the patient with a detailed report of the findings and recommended follow-up. This chapter will discuss the importance of follow-up after a colonoscopy, the recommended follow-up schedule, and what to expect during follow-up appointments.

The primary reason for follow-up after a colonoscopy is to ensure that any abnormalities detected during the procedure are monitored and treated if necessary. Abnormal findings may include the presence of polyps, which are small growths that can develop on the inner lining of the colon. While most polyps are benign, some can become cancerous if left untreated. Additionally, follow-up is necessary if biopsies were taken during the procedure, as these can reveal abnormalities that require further investigation or treatment.

The recommended follow-up schedule for colonoscopy varies depending on the findings and the patient's individual risk factors. In general, patients with a normal colonoscopy can wait ten years before their next screening. However, patients with abnormal findings may require more frequent follow-up appointments. For example, patients with one or two small, low-risk polyps may need a follow-up colonoscopy in three to five years, while those with larger or more high-risk polyps may need a repeat colonoscopy in one to three years. Patients who have had colorectal cancer or a family history of the disease may require more frequent colonoscopies or other screening tests.

During follow-up appointments, the doctor will review the results of the colonoscopy and any biopsies taken during the procedure. They may also perform a physical exam, discuss any symptoms the patient may be experiencing, and provide recommendations for future screenings. If abnormalities were detected during the colonoscopy, the doctor may recommend further testing or treatment, such as additional imaging tests, surgery, or medication.

In addition to following the recommended screening schedule, patients can take steps to reduce their risk of developing colon and rectal cancer. Maintaining a healthy diet that is high in fruits, vegetables, and whole grains and low in processed foods and red meat can help reduce the risk of developing polyps and cancer. Regular exercise can also lower the risk of colorectal cancer, as can avoiding smoking and excessive alcohol consumption.

Patients should also be aware of the symptoms of colorectal cancer, which can include changes in bowel habits, blood in the stool, abdominal pain or cramping, and unexplained weight loss. If any of these symptoms occur, patients should contact their doctor right away, even if they are not due for a follow-up colonoscopy.

What other tests are available to evaluate the colon?

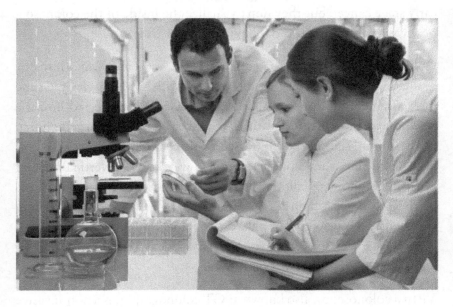

Colon cancer is the third most common cancer in the United States, and the second leading cause of cancer deaths. It is important to detect colon cancer early, as it is much more treatable in its early stages. There are several tests available to evaluate the colon, each with its own advantages and disadvantages.

Fecal Occult Blood Test (FOBT) and Fecal Immunochemical Test (FIT) are two of the most common tests used to screen for colon cancer. Both tests check for blood in the stool, which can be an early sign of colon cancer or polyps. FOBT is a test that is done at home, where the patient collects small samples of their stool on special cards or in a container. The samples are then sent to a laboratory for analysis. FIT is similar, but it uses a different method to detect blood in the stool. It requires only one stool sample and is more specific for detecting cancer. Both tests are non-invasive and can be done easily at home, and they have a high sensitivity for detecting polyps and early stage cancer, but they don't visualize the inside of the colon, so a positive result will require a follow-up colonoscopy.

Colonoscopy is the most common and most accurate test for evaluating the colon. It is a procedure in which a long, flexible tube with a camera on the end (called a colonoscope) is inserted into the rectum and moved through the large intestine to examine the lining of the colon. The procedure is used to detect colon cancer, as well as other conditions such as inflammatory bowel disease, diverticulitis, and polyps. Colonoscopy allows the doctor to look directly at the inside of the colon, take biopsies, and remove any polyps that are found. It is considered the gold standard for colon cancer screening, but it does have some disadvantages. It is invasive, it requires sedation or anesthesia, and it can be uncomfortable.

Virtual colonoscopy, also known as CT colonography, is a non-invasive test that uses a CT scan to create detailed images of the inside of the colon. The patient is given a laxative to clean out the colon, and then they lie on a table while a CT scanner takes pictures of the inside of the colon. The images are then analyzed by a radiologist to look for any abnormalities. Virtual colonoscopy is less invasive than traditional colonoscopy, and it does not require sedation or anesthesia, but it is not as accurate and it doesn't allow for polyp removal.

Sigmoidoscopy is similar to colonoscopy, but it only examines the lower part of the colon, known as the sigmoid colon and the rectum. It uses a shorter and more flexible scope called a sigmoidoscope and is done with sedation. It is a less invasive test than colonoscopy, but it doesn't visualize the entire colon.

Barium enema is a test that involves injecting a chalky liquid called barium into the rectum and colon through a tube, then using X-rays to create images of the colon. The barium coats the inside of the colon, making any abnormalities visible on the X-ray. It is considered less accurate than colonoscopy and it has been largely replaced by virtual colonoscopy.

DNA stool tests are a newer type of test that looks for specific genetic mutations that can indicate colon cancer. It is a non-invasive test that requires only a small sample of stool, which is then analyzed in a laboratory for the presence of certain genetic markers. It is more specific for detecting colon cancer than FOBT or FIT.

Alternative Colorectal Cancer Screening Methods

Colorectal cancer is the third most common cancer diagnosed in both men and women worldwide. Screening for colorectal cancer can detect precancerous polyps or early cancer, allowing for early intervention and improved outcomes. Colonoscopy is considered the gold standard for colorectal cancer screening, but there are other screening methods available as well. Below we will discuss some of the alternative screening methods for colorectal cancer and their benefits and limitations.

Fecal Immunochemical Test (FIT)

FIT is a stool-based test that detects the presence of blood in the stool. It is a simple and non-invasive test that can be performed at home. Patients collect a stool sample and send it to a laboratory for analysis. FIT is recommended to be done once a year.

The advantage of FIT is its simplicity and non-invasiveness. However, FIT has a relatively low sensitivity for detecting precancerous polyps and early-stage cancer. Furthermore, FIT only detects blood in the stool and cannot identify the source of bleeding. False-positive results can also occur due to non-cancerous causes, such as hemorrhoids or inflammatory bowel disease.

Stool DNA Test

Stool DNA testing is another non-invasive test that can be performed at home. It detects abnormal DNA changes in the cells shed into the stool. This test is recommended to be done every three years.

The advantage of stool DNA testing is its higher sensitivity than FIT for detecting precancerous polyps and early-stage cancer. Additionally, stool DNA testing can detect abnormalities in specific genes associated with colorectal cancer, providing additional information that FIT cannot. However, stool DNA testing is more expensive than FIT, and false-positive results can also occur.

Flexible Sigmoidoscopy

Flexible sigmoidoscopy is an invasive procedure that involves inserting a flexible tube with a camera into the rectum and lower colon. It allows for visualization of the rectum and sigmoid colon and can detect precancerous polyps or early cancer. It is recommended to be done every five years.

The advantage of flexible sigmoidoscopy is its ability to detect precancerous polyps and early cancer in the lower colon. It is also less invasive than colonoscopy and does not require the same level of bowel preparation. However, flexible sigmoidoscopy only examines the lower part of the colon, so it cannot detect abnormalities in the upper colon. Additionally, if an abnormality is found during the procedure, a follow-up colonoscopy may be required.

Computed Tomography (CT) Colonography

CT colonography, also known as virtual colonoscopy, is a non-invasive test that uses X-rays and computer technology to create detailed images of the colon. It is recommended to be done every five years.

The advantage of CT colonography is its ability to detect precancerous polyps and early-stage cancer. It is also less invasive than colonoscopy and does not require sedation. Additionally, CT colonography can visualize the entire colon and can identify other abnormalities, such as diverticulitis or inflammatory bowel disease. However, bowel preparation is still required, and if an abnormality is found during the procedure, a follow-up colonoscopy may be required.

Blood Tests

Blood tests are not a primary screening method for colorectal cancer, but they can be used to help detect the disease in certain circumstances. For example, if a patient has symptoms of colorectal cancer, a blood test can be used to check for anemia, which may be a sign of bleeding in the digestive tract. Additionally, certain blood tests can be used to monitor treatment or recurrence of colorectal cancer.

Fecal Occult Blood Test

Fecal Occult Blood Test (FOBT) is a screening test that is used to detect the presence of blood in the stool, which could be a sign of colorectal cancer or other gastrointestinal conditions. The test is simple, non-invasive, and can be done at home. Below we will discuss what the FOBT is, how it works, and its benefits and limitations as an alternative to colonoscopy.

FOBT is a type of medical test that analyzes stool samples for the presence of blood. It is called "occult" because the blood in the stool may not be visible to the naked eye, and the test is used to detect small amounts of blood that may not be visible during a routine physical examination. The test is recommended as a screening tool for colorectal cancer in people over the age of 50.

The FOBT test works by detecting small amounts of blood in the stool. The test kit usually comes with instructions on how to collect the stool sample at home. The sample is then sent to a laboratory for analysis. The laboratory analyzes the sample for the presence of blood, which could be a sign of cancer or other gastrointestinal conditions.

1. There are two types of FOBT tests: the guaiac-based FOBT (gFOBT) and the fecal immunochemical test (FIT). The gFOBT test uses a chemical called guaiac to detect the presence of blood in the stool. The FIT test uses antibodies to detect blood in the stool. The FIT test is considered more accurate and easier to use than the gFOBT test.

FOBT has several benefits as an alternative to colonoscopy. It is non-invasive, which means it does not require sedation or anesthesia. The test is also relatively inexpensive and can be done at home, which is convenient for people who cannot or do not want to undergo colonoscopy. Additionally, FOBT can detect small amounts of blood in the stool, which can help detect colorectal cancer in its early stages.

However, FOBT also has some limitations. The test is not as accurate as colonoscopy in detecting colorectal cancer or polyps. FOBT can also produce false-positive results, which means the test may detect blood in the stool even when there is no cancer or other gastrointestinal condition present. False-positive results can lead to unnecessary follow-up tests and procedures, which can cause anxiety and discomfort.

It is important to note that FOBT should not be used as a replacement for colonoscopy in all cases. Colonoscopy is still considered the gold standard for detecting and preventing colorectal cancer. However, FOBT can be a good alternative for people who cannot or do not want to undergo colonoscopy.

Fecal Immunochemical Test

Fecal immunochemical tests (FIT) are a type of screening test used to detect the presence of blood in the stool, which can be a sign of colorectal cancer or other gastrointestinal conditions. FITs are an alternative to colonoscopy for individuals who may not be able to undergo the procedure, or who may prefer a less invasive option. Below we will explore the use of FITs, how they work, their benefits and limitations, and how they compare to other colorectal cancer screening methods.

FITs are designed to detect the presence of blood in the stool that may not be visible to the naked eye. This type of test uses antibodies to detect hemoglobin, a protein found in red blood cells. The test is performed using a small sample of stool, which is collected at home and sent to a laboratory for analysis. The laboratory then analyzes the sample for the presence of blood using a chemical reaction with the antibodies.

One of the main benefits of FITs is their non-invasive nature. Unlike a colonoscopy, which involves inserting a camera into the colon, FITs can be done at home with minimal discomfort. Additionally, FITs are more cost-effective than colonoscopy and can be a good option for individuals who may not be able to undergo the procedure due to medical conditions, such as a bleeding disorder or history of heart disease.

However, FITs also have some limitations. One of the main limitations is their accuracy. While FITs are designed to detect the presence of blood, they may not be able to distinguish between blood from cancerous or non-cancerous sources. Additionally, FITs are not able to detect polyps, which can also be a sign of colorectal cancer. For this reason, individuals who receive a positive result on a FIT will typically be referred for further testing, such as a colonoscopy.

Another limitation of FITs is that they require regular testing. The American Cancer Society recommends that individuals with average risk of colorectal cancer begin screening at age 45 and continue until age 75. FITs should be performed every year, while colonoscopies are typically recommended every 10 years for individuals with a normal risk.

Compared to other colorectal cancer screening methods, FITs have both advantages and disadvantages. Compared to colonoscopy, FITs are less invasive and have a lower risk of complications. However, colonoscopy is more accurate in detecting polyps and can also be used to remove them during the procedure. In addition, a colonoscopy can be used to diagnose and treat other gastrointestinal conditions, such as inflammatory bowel disease.

Other screening methods include stool DNA tests, which are similar to FITs but can also detect genetic mutations associated with colorectal cancer, and virtual colonoscopy, which uses a CT scan to produce images of the colon. Each screening method has its own benefits and limitations, and the choice of which test to use will depend on the individual's personal preferences and medical history.

CT Colonography

CT colonography, also known as virtual colonoscopy, is a screening test that uses computed tomography (CT) technology to produce detailed images of the colon and rectum. Unlike traditional colonoscopy, which involves the insertion of a flexible tube with a camera into the rectum, CT colonography is non-invasive and requires no sedation. Below we will discuss the process of CT colonography, its benefits and limitations, and how it compares to traditional colonoscopy.

The Process of CT Colonography:

Prior to the procedure, patients are required to follow a specific diet and bowel preparation instructions to ensure that the colon is empty and free of any stool or debris. During the procedure, the patient lies on a table and a small tube is inserted into the rectum to inflate the colon with air. This allows for better visualization of the colon walls and any abnormalities. The patient is then moved through a CT scanner, which takes multiple images of the colon. The images are then combined to create a three-dimensional virtual image of the colon that can be examined by a radiologist for abnormalities such as polyps or tumors.

Benefits of CT Colonography:

CT colonography has several advantages over traditional colonoscopy. Firstly, it is a non-invasive procedure that does not require sedation or the use of a scope. This can be particularly beneficial for patients who are unable or unwilling to undergo traditional colonoscopy due to the discomfort or risk of complications. Additionally, CT colonography is quicker than traditional colonoscopy and does not require a recovery period. Patients can return to their daily activities immediately after the procedure. Lastly, CT colonography has been shown to be effective in detecting colon cancer and precancerous polyps, particularly those that are larger than 1 cm.

Limitations of CT Colonography:

While CT colonography has many benefits, it also has some limitations. The most significant limitation is that it is less accurate in detecting small polyps than traditional colonoscopy. Additionally, CT colonography may not be suitable for patients who have a history of abdominal surgery or other conditions that may make it difficult to inflate the colon with air. Lastly, CT colonography requires a higher radiation dose than traditional colonoscopy, which may be a concern for some patients.

Comparison to Traditional Colonoscopy:

CT colonography and traditional colonoscopy have different strengths and weaknesses. Traditional colonoscopy is generally considered the gold standard for detecting colon cancer and polyps as it allows for direct visualization and the removal of any abnormalities. However, it is an invasive procedure that requires sedation and has a small risk of complications such as bleeding or perforation. On the other hand, CT colonography is non-invasive and has a lower risk of complications. However, it may be less accurate in detecting small polyps and requires a higher radiation dose.

Pediatric Colonoscopy

Pediatric colonoscopy is a procedure used to examine the colon and rectum in children. It is similar to the adult colonoscopy but with some differences. The procedure is usually performed under sedation or general anesthesia, and it involves using a colonoscope, a long, flexible tube with a camera at the end, to visualize the colon and rectum.

Pediatric colonoscopy is used for various diagnostic and therapeutic purposes. Some of the common indications include abdominal pain, rectal bleeding, diarrhea, constipation, and suspected inflammatory bowel disease (IBD). Other indications include the evaluation of polyps, screening for colorectal cancer, and the management of gastrointestinal bleeding.

Pediatric colonoscopy is a safe and effective procedure, but it requires careful preparation and monitoring. The preparation for the procedure is similar to that of adults, but the bowel preparation solutions used may be different. The child may need to follow a special diet before the procedure, and laxatives may be used to clear the colon of stool.

During the procedure, the child is usually placed under sedation or general anesthesia to help them relax and prevent any discomfort or pain. The colonoscope is then inserted through the rectum and advanced through the colon while the doctor views the images on a monitor. Biopsies or polyp removal may be done during the procedure if necessary.

After the procedure, the child may need to stay in the recovery room for a short period until the sedation wears off. The child may experience some mild discomfort, bloating, or gas after the procedure, but these symptoms usually resolve quickly. The doctor will provide instructions on resuming normal activities, including when the child can eat and drink again.

Pediatric colonoscopy is generally safe, but like any medical procedure, it has some risks. The risks may include bleeding, infection, perforation of the colon, and reactions to sedation or anesthesia. However, these risks are rare, and most children recover well after the procedure.

Pediatric colonoscopy is an important diagnostic and therapeutic tool that can help identify and treat various gastrointestinal conditions in children. It is particularly useful in evaluating inflammatory bowel disease, which can be difficult to diagnose in children. The procedure can also help detect and remove polyps, which can be a precursor to colorectal cancer.

Alternative screening methods for colorectal cancer, such as fecal occult blood tests or CT colonography, are generally not recommended for pediatric patients. These tests are designed for adults and may not be appropriate or effective for children.

Indications and Preparation

Colonoscopy is a medical procedure that involves the examination of the colon or large intestine, and it is commonly used to identify and diagnose various conditions such as colorectal cancer, inflammatory bowel disease, and polyps. Although colonoscopy is typically performed on adults, there are certain situations where it may be necessary for children to undergo the procedure as well. Below we will discuss the indications for pediatric colonoscopy and the preparation that is required for this procedure.

Indications for Pediatric Colonoscopy:

There are several reasons why a pediatrician may recommend a colonoscopy for a child. One of the most common indications is the presence of gastrointestinal symptoms such as chronic diarrhea, abdominal pain, and rectal bleeding. These symptoms may indicate a number of conditions, including inflammatory bowel disease, celiac disease, and colon polyps. In some cases, a colonoscopy may also be recommended as a diagnostic tool for children who have a family history of colorectal cancer or other genetic conditions that increase their risk of developing this type of cancer.

Another indication for pediatric colonoscopy is the detection of blood in the stool. This may be a sign of inflammation or damage to the lining of the colon or rectum, or it could be an indication of more serious conditions such as ulcerative colitis or Crohn's disease. In some cases, a colonoscopy may also be used to investigate the cause of anemia in a child, which could be due to bleeding in the gastrointestinal tract.

Finally, pediatric colonoscopy may be indicated for the removal of polyps. While colon polyps are relatively rare in children, they can occur and may require removal to prevent further complications.

Preparation for Pediatric Colonoscopy:

The preparation for pediatric colonoscopy is similar to that of adults, although there are some key differences. Before the procedure, the child will need to undergo a bowel cleanse, which involves the consumption of a special solution that helps to clear the colon of any stool or debris. The solution is usually given in several doses, and the child will need to drink a lot of fluids to stay hydrated.

In addition to the bowel cleanse, the child may need to fast for several hours before the procedure. This is typically done to ensure that the stomach and intestines are empty, which makes it easier for the doctor to see the colon during the procedure. The child may also need to avoid certain foods and medications in the days leading up to the procedure, as directed by their doctor.

During the Procedure:

During the colonoscopy, the child will be sedated to help them relax and minimize any discomfort or pain. The doctor will insert a flexible tube with a small camera on the end, called a colonoscope, into the child's rectum and slowly guide it through the colon. The camera allows the doctor to see the inside of the colon and identify any abnormalities or polyps.

If polyps are detected, the doctor may remove them during the procedure using special instruments passed through the colonoscope. In some cases, a biopsy may also be taken to help diagnose a condition or determine the nature of an abnormality.

After the Procedure:

Following the colonoscopy, the child will need to be monitored for a short period of time until the sedative wears off. They may feel bloated or have some discomfort in the abdomen for a few hours, but this typically resolves on its own.

It is important to follow the doctor's instructions for recovery, which may include avoiding certain foods or activities for a period of time. The doctor will also discuss the results of the colonoscopy with the child and their parent or caregiver, and recommend any further treatment or monitoring if necessary.

Innovations in Colonoscopy Technology

Colonoscopy is a vital diagnostic tool for detecting abnormalities in the colon and rectum, including polyps and cancer. The procedure involves inserting a long, flexible tube with a camera and light source into the colon through the rectum, allowing the doctor to examine the lining of the colon and potentially remove any polyps detected. Over the years, advancements in technology have greatly improved the accuracy and effectiveness of colonoscopies, making them even more essential in the early detection and prevention of colorectal cancer.

One of the most significant technological advances in colonoscopy is the development of high-definition imaging systems. These systems allow for clearer, more detailed images of the colon and rectum, which can help doctors identify even small polyps or abnormalities that may have been missed with older imaging technology. High-definition imaging also allows for better visualization of the colon's anatomy, which can help doctors navigate through it more easily and safely.

Another recent innovation in colonoscopy technology is the use of narrow-band imaging (NBI). NBI is an optical filter technology that uses specific light wavelengths to enhance the contrast between the blood vessels and surrounding tissues in the colon. This makes it easier for doctors to identify and differentiate between normal and abnormal tissue in the colon, and can potentially reduce the need for unnecessary biopsies.

Virtual colonoscopy, or computed tomography (CT) colonography, is another emerging technology in the field of colonoscopy. This non-invasive imaging technique uses specialized X-ray equipment and computer software to create detailed 3D images of the colon and rectum. Virtual colonoscopy can be used to detect polyps and other abnormalities, but does not allow for their removal during the procedure. While virtual colonoscopy may be a good option for some patients, it is not yet widely available and may not be covered by all insurance plans.

Another promising innovation in colonoscopy technology is the development of capsule endoscopy. This is a non-invasive procedure that involves swallowing a small, wireless camera capsule that travels through the digestive system and captures images of the colon and rectum. Once the capsule is excreted, the images are downloaded and analyzed by a doctor. While capsule endoscopy is still in the early stages of development, it has the potential to be a less invasive and more patient-friendly alternative to traditional colonoscopy.

Despite the numerous advancements in colonoscopy technology, the procedure does still carry some risks, including bleeding and perforation. However, these risks are generally very low, and the benefits of early detection and prevention of colorectal cancer far outweigh the risks for most patients. Additionally, technological advancements have helped to minimize these risks even further.

High-Definition Colonoscopy

High-definition colonoscopy is a relatively new technology that has revolutionized the way doctors perform colonoscopies. A colonoscopy is a medical procedure used to examine the colon and rectum for signs of disease or cancer. The procedure involves inserting a flexible tube with a camera into the rectum, and then advancing it through the colon. The camera transmits images of the inside of the colon to a monitor, which the doctor uses to examine the colon for abnormalities. High-definition colonoscopy uses state-of-the-art technology to provide clearer, more detailed images of the inside of the colon, making it easier for doctors to identify and remove polyps and other abnormalities.

High-definition colonoscopy is performed using a high-definition colonoscope, which is a type of endoscope that has a high-definition video camera attached to it. The camera captures detailed, high-quality images of the inside of the colon, which are then displayed on a high-definition monitor. The images produced by a high-definition colonoscope are much sharper and clearer than those produced by a traditional colonoscope, which uses standard-definition technology.

One of the main benefits of high-definition colonoscopy is that it improves the detection of polyps and other abnormalities in the colon. Polyps are small growths that can develop on the lining of the colon. While most polyps are benign, some can become cancerous over time. Identifying and removing polyps during a colonoscopy is an important way to prevent colon cancer. High-definition colonoscopy improves the detection of polyps by providing clearer, more detailed images of the inside of the colon. This makes it easier for doctors to identify and remove small or flat polyps, which can be difficult to see with a traditional colonoscope.

Another benefit of high-definition colonoscopy is that it reduces the need for repeat procedures. When a polyp is identified during a colonoscopy, it is typically removed during the same procedure. However, if the doctor is unable to fully remove the polyp or if there are other concerns, a repeat procedure may be necessary. High-definition colonoscopy reduces the need for repeat procedures by improving the detection and removal of polyps during the initial procedure.

High-definition colonoscopy is also less invasive than traditional colonoscopy. The high-definition colonoscope is designed to be more flexible and maneuverable than a traditional colonoscope, which makes it easier for the doctor to navigate through the colon. This reduces the risk of injury to the colon and makes the procedure more comfortable for the patient.

Despite its many benefits, high-definition colonoscopy is not yet widely available. It requires specialized equipment and training, which can make it more expensive than traditional colonoscopy. Additionally, not all doctors are trained in the use of high-definition colonoscopy, which can limit patient access to the technology.

Narrow Band Imaging

Narrow Band Imaging (NBI) is a modern technology used in colonoscopy to improve visualization of the colon mucosa. It is a non-invasive procedure that utilizes narrow-band filters to enhance the image quality of the mucosal surface. NBI is an advanced tool that helps physicians to identify any potential abnormalities, including polyps, adenomas, or even early-stage cancers, that may be present in the colon. Below we will discuss how Narrow Band Imaging works and its benefits in improving the accuracy and efficacy of colonoscopy.

The traditional colonoscopy procedure involves the use of white light to visualize the mucosal surface of the colon. However, this technique has limitations, especially when it comes to detecting subtle changes in the colon's lining. Narrow Band Imaging overcomes these limitations by using narrow-band filters that enhance the visualization of the colon mucosa.

The NBI system utilizes blue and green lights to enhance the contrast of the colon's lining. The blue light penetrates the surface of the colon mucosa, while the green light is reflected off the mucosa's surface. This creates a high-contrast image that highlights the subtle differences in the colon's lining, making it easier for the physician to identify any potential abnormalities.

The use of Narrow Band Imaging has several benefits over traditional colonoscopy. Firstly, it allows physicians to better differentiate between different tissue types. This can help them to identify polyps and adenomas that may be missed using traditional colonoscopy techniques. Additionally, NBI can help to identify areas of inflammation or other abnormalities that may require further investigation.

One of the main benefits of NBI is its ability to detect small polyps that may be difficult to visualize using traditional colonoscopy techniques. Studies have shown that NBI can improve the detection rate of small polyps by up to 70%. This is particularly important as small polyps are often missed during traditional colonoscopy procedures and can develop into cancer over time.

Another benefit of NBI is its ability to improve the accuracy of colonoscopy procedures. The high-contrast images provided by NBI allow physicians to make more accurate diagnoses and reduce the need for further investigations. This can help to improve patient outcomes and reduce healthcare costs.

Narrow Band Imaging is a safe and non-invasive procedure that can be performed in conjunction with traditional colonoscopy. The procedure does not require any special preparation or additional procedures, and patients can usually resume their normal activities immediately after the procedure.

However, there are some limitations to NBI. The procedure is not effective for patients with severe bowel inflammation or those who have had previous bowel surgery. Additionally, NBI is not suitable for detecting certain types of polyps, such as sessile serrated polyps.

Artificial Intelligence

Artificial intelligence (AI) is a rapidly advancing technology that has the potential to revolutionize many aspects of healthcare, including colonoscopy. Colonoscopy is a commonly used procedure to screen for colorectal cancer and other gastrointestinal conditions. It involves the use of a flexible scope with a camera and light to visualize the colon and rectum. The use of AI in colonoscopy can aid in the detection of polyps, improve accuracy, and reduce the risk of missed lesions.

One of the key benefits of using AI in colonoscopy is its ability to detect polyps. Polyps are abnormal growths in the colon that can be precursors to colorectal cancer. The detection of polyps during colonoscopy is important because they can be removed before they become cancerous. However, polyps can be difficult to detect, particularly when they are small or located in hard-to-see areas of the colon. AI can aid in the detection of polyps by analyzing the images captured during colonoscopy and highlighting areas that may be indicative of a polyp. This can help to improve the accuracy of colonoscopy and reduce the risk of missed lesions.

Another advantage of using AI in colonoscopy is its ability to improve accuracy. Colonoscopy is a highly operator-dependent procedure, and the accuracy of the procedure can vary depending on the skill and experience of the endoscopist. AI can provide real-time feedback to the endoscopist during the procedure, highlighting areas that may be missed or require additional attention. This can help to ensure that the entire colon is thoroughly examined and can improve the accuracy of the procedure.

AI can also aid in the diagnosis of other gastrointestinal conditions. For example, AI algorithms can be used to analyze the images captured during colonoscopy to detect signs of inflammatory bowel disease (IBD) or other conditions such as diverticulitis. This can help to ensure that patients receive timely and accurate diagnoses, which can lead to more effective treatment and improved outcomes.

However, there are also challenges associated with the use of AI in colonoscopy. One of the main challenges is the development of accurate and reliable algorithms. AI algorithms require large datasets to be trained, and the accuracy of the algorithm depends on the quality and size of the dataset. In addition, the use of AI in colonoscopy requires sophisticated computer hardware and software, which can be expensive and may require specialized training.

Another challenge is the integration of AI into the existing workflow of colonoscopy. The use of AI may require additional time and resources, and it may be difficult to integrate AI into existing clinical workflows. Additionally, there may be concerns about the impact of AI on the role of the endoscopist, and there may be resistance to the adoption of new technologies in some healthcare settings.

Despite these challenges, the potential benefits of using AI in colonoscopy are significant. The use of AI can aid in the detection of polyps, improve accuracy, and aid in the diagnosis of other gastrointestinal conditions. As AI technology continues to evolve, it is likely that its role in colonoscopy will become increasingly important. However, careful consideration must be given to the development, implementation, and integration of AI into clinical practice to ensure that its benefits are realized and that patient safety is not compromised.

Other FAQ

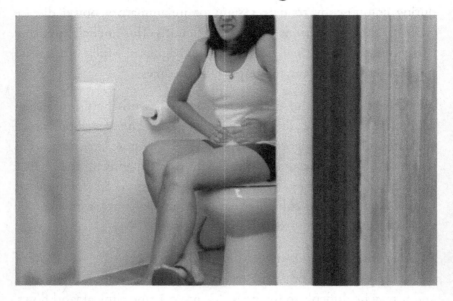

What is a Colonoscopy?

A Colonoscopy is a routine medical procedure, usually performed as a preventative measure against colon cancer. The procedure involves inserting a long, flexible tube into the rectum and colon, and inflated with air to allow the doctor to get a clear view of the inside of the colon.

Most people report that the procedure is not painful, although there may be some discomfort from the air being inflated into the colon. The whole procedure usually takes less than an hour. After the procedure, the patient will be able to go home and resume their normal activities.

Do they put you to sleep for a colonoscopy?

A colonoscopy is a medical procedure that allows your doctor to look at the inside of your large intestine (also called the colon) and rectum. The procedure is done using a long, thin tube called a colonoscope.

A colonoscopy is usually done in a hospital or outpatient center. You will be asked to lie on your side on a table. Your doctor will insert the colonoscope into your rectum and then slowly guide it through your large intestine.

If you are having a colonoscopy, you will be given a sedative to help you relax. You may also be given a pain reliever. You will be awake during the procedure, but you will not be able to feel any pain.

The entire procedure takes about 30 minutes. Once the colonoscope is in place, your doctor will be able to see the inside of your large intestine. If necessary, your doctor may take a biopsy (a small tissue sample) during the procedure.

After the procedure is finished, the colonoscope will be removed and you will be taken to a recovery area where you will be monitored for a short time.

How long will it take to recover from a colonoscopy?

A colonoscopy is a medical procedure used to examine the large intestine, or colon. The colon is the last part of the digestive system, and the procedure is used to identify any problems with the colon, such as polyps, ulcers, or cancer.

The colonoscopy procedure itself is relatively quick, and most people report feeling little to no pain during the procedure. However, the recovery process can take a bit longer. Most people feel some discomfort and bloating immediately after the procedure, and it is not uncommon to experience cramping, gas, and diarrhea. These symptoms usually last for 24-48 hours.

It is important to drink plenty of fluids and eat a light diet following a colonoscopy to help ease these symptoms. Avoiding dairy and high-fiber foods is often recommended, as they can contribute to diarrhea. It is also important to take it easy and avoid strenuous activity for a day or two following the procedure, as this can also aggravate symptoms.

Overall, the recovery from a colonoscopy is generally not too difficult, and most people feel back to normal within a few days. However, if you have any concerns or your symptoms are severe, be sure to talk to your doctor.

Is colonoscopy a painful procedure?

Colonoscopy is a procedure that is used to evaluate the large intestine (colon) for conditions such as Crohn's disease, ulcerative colitis, Diverticulitis, and colon cancer. The colonoscopy procedure involves the insertion of a long, flexible, lighted tube (colonoscope) into the rectum. The colonoscope is then advanced through the entire length of the large intestine, and the lining of the colon is examined.

Some people may experience some discomfort during the colonoscopy procedure, but it is generally not a painful procedure. The colonoscope is inserted into the rectum, which is the end of the large intestine. The rectum is a short, muscular tube that is about four inches long and connects the large intestine to the anus. The rectum contains a small amount of liquid, which lubricates the colonoscope as it is inserted.

As the colonoscope is advanced through the large intestine, air is injected through the colonoscope to inflate the intestine and give the doctor a better view. This may cause some cramping or bloating. Some people may also experience a feeling of fullness or pressure.

The colonoscope also has a camera attached to it, which allows the doctor to see the lining of the colon. The doctor may biopsy (take a small sample of) the lining of the colon if anything abnormal is seen. The biopsy is usually not painful, but some people may experience a cramping sensation.

The entire colonoscopy procedure usually takes 30-60 minutes. After the procedure, most people can go home and resume their normal activities.

What exactly happens during a colonoscopy?

A colonoscopy is a medical procedure that allows a doctor to examine the lining of the large intestine (colon) and rectum. A thin, flexible tube called a colonoscope is used to view the inside of the colon.

The colonoscope has a light and a camera lens at its tip. The doctor guide the colonoscope through the colon, taking pictures along the way. If anything abnormal is found, the doctor may remove a small tissue sample (biopsy) for further examination.

A colonoscopy usually takes 30 to 60 minutes. During the procedure, the person will lie on their side on an exam table. The doctor will insert the colonoscope into the person's rectum.

The colonoscope will then be slowly guided through the colon. The person may be asked to move into different positions to help the doctor get a better view. As the colonoscope moves along, the doctor will pump air into the colon to help keep the colonoscope afloat and prevent it from hitting the colon wall too hard.

The colonoscope has a light and a tiny video camera at its tip. The doctor guide the colonoscope through the colon, taking pictures along the way. If anything abnormal is found, the doctor may remove a small tissue sample (biopsy) for further examination.

How long does a colonoscopy take?

A colonoscopy usually takes 30 to 60 minutes. During the procedure, the person will lie on their side on an exam table. The doctor will insert the colonoscope into the person's rectum.

The colonoscope will then be slowly guided through the colon. The person may be asked to move into different positions to help the doctor get a better view. As the colonoscope moves along, the doctor will pump air into the colon to help keep the colonoscope afloat and prevent it from hitting the colon wall too hard.

How long do you stay in hospital after a colonoscopy?

How long you stay in hospital after a colonoscopy depends on the results of the procedure itself. If everything goes well and no polyps or other abnormalities are found, you may be able to go home the same day. If polyps are found, they will be removed during the colonoscopy. Recovery from this take a little longer, and you may be required to stay overnight for observation. In rare cases, more serious problems may be found that require surgery. This would obviously extended your stay in hospital.

Overall, the length of time you stay in hospital after a colonoscopy is relatively short. The procedure itself only takes a few minutes, and even if polyps are found and removed, you should be able to go home the same day or the day after. In very rare cases, you may need to stay longer if complications arise, but this is not the norm. So, while you may be a little anxious about the procedure, you can rest assured that it won't take up too much of your time.

How will I feel day after colonoscopy?

Most people feel great after a colonoscopy. The prep can be pretty intense, but it's worth it to get a clean bill of health. Here's what you can expect in the days following your procedure.

You may have some cramping and bloating for the first day or so. This is normal and should go away within a day or two. You may also have some gas and increased bowel movements for a few days. This is also normal and should resolve itself soon.

If you had sedation for your procedure, you may feel groggy for the rest of the day. You should not operate heavy machinery or drive for the rest of the day. You may also have trouble remembering things for the rest of the day. This is all normal and will go away soon.

Drinking plenty of fluids is important after a colonoscopy. This will help replace the fluids you lost during the prep and will help prevent dehydration. You should also avoid alcohol for 24 hours after the procedure.

You should be able to return to your normal activities the day after your colonoscopy. If you have any questions or concerns, be sure to follow up with your doctor.

Do they put you to sleep for a colonoscopy?

Although a colonoscopy is not a particularly long or invasive procedure, many people are still nervous about undergoing one. A common question that people have is whether or not they will be put to sleep for the procedure.

The answer to this question is that it depends on the person and the preference of the doctor. In some cases, the doctor may feel that it is necessary to put the patient under anesthesia in order to complete the colonoscopy successfully. Other times, the doctor may be able to perform the procedure while the patient is awake and sedated.

If the doctor does decide to put the patient under anesthesia, they will be given a general anesthetic. This will put them into a deep sleep for the duration of the procedure. The anesthetic can be given through an IV or with a gas mask.

Once the anesthetic has taken effect, the doctor will begin the colonoscopy. The patient will not be aware of anything during this time. Once the procedure is completed, the anesthetic will be turned off and the patient will wake up.

If the doctor decides to keep the patient awake, they will be given a sedative through an IV. This will help to relax them and make them feel drowsy. The sedative will not put them into a deep sleep, but it will make them less aware of what is going on around them.

The doctor will then begin the colonoscopy. The patient may be aware of some pressure or discomfort, but they should not be in any pain. If they do start to feel pain, the doctor will give them more of the sedative.

Once the procedure is completed, the sedative will be turned off and the patient will be allowed to wake up. They may feel a little groggy and disoriented, but this will quickly wear off.

In most cases, the decision of whether or not to put the patient under anesthesia is up to the doctor. However, the patient may be able to request one or the other. It is important to discuss all of the options with the doctor before the procedure so that you can make the best decision for yourself.

Why have a colonoscopy?

A colonoscopy is an important procedure that can help to diagnosis and treat many different gastrointestinal disorders. It is a safe and effective procedure that is generally well-tolerated by patients. While there are some potential risks and complications associated with colonoscopy, these are usually minor and can be effectively managed by experienced healthcare providers.

A colonoscopy is used to detect changes in the large intestine and rectum. It is also used to remove polyps, which are growths on the lining of the intestines. The doctor performing the colonoscopy will use a thin, flexible tube with a light and a camera attached to it. The camera will send images to a monitor, where the doctor can look for anything abnormal. In order to prepare for a colonoscopy, the patient will be asked to follow a strict diet and to take a laxative. The day before the procedure, the patient will also be asked to not eat or drink anything after midnight.

How long will it take to recover from a colonoscopy?

A colonoscopy is a medical procedure used to visualise the large intestine and detect any abnormalities. It is carried out using a thin, flexible telescope called a colonoscope, which is inserted into the rectum and passed through the entire length of the colon.

The procedure itself usually takes around 30 minutes, but the total time from arrival at the hospital to discharge can be several hours. This is because the colon needs to be thoroughly cleansed before the procedure can take place, and this can take a few hours.

Most people feel some discomfort during the procedure, but this is usually mild and goes away quickly. Some people may experience some cramping or bloating afterwards, but this usually improves within a day or so.

It is important to drink plenty of fluids and eat a light diet for the first day or two after the procedure to help the digestive system recover. People should also avoid strenuous activity for a few days.

In most cases, people can return to their normal activities the day after the procedure.

Is colonoscopy a painful procedure?

A colonoscopy is a medical procedure used to diagnose and treat various conditions of the large intestine, including cancer. The colon, or large intestine, is a long, coiled tube that starts at the small intestine and ends at the rectum.

During a colonoscopy, a long, flexible tube, called a colonoscope, is inserted into the rectum and advanced through the entire length of the colon. The colonoscope has a light and a camera at its tip, which allows the doctor to see the inside of the colon. Biopsies (removal of small tissue samples) and polyp removal can be done during a colonoscopy.

A colonoscopy is generally a safe procedure with a low risk of complications. However, as with any medical procedure, there are some risks associated with colonoscopy. These risks include:

- Bleeding

- Infection

- Perforation (a hole in the wall of the intestine)

- Reaction to the sedative used during the procedure

Most people do not experience any pain during a colonoscopy. However, some people may experience mild discomfort, such as cramping or bloating, during the procedure.

If a biopsy is taken or a polyp is removed during the colonoscopy, you may experience some bleeding from the site. This bleeding is usually minor and stops on its own. However, if the bleeding is more than a teaspoonful, or if it lasts for more than a few minutes, you should call your doctor.

There is a small risk of infection associated with colonoscopy. This risk can be increased if the colonoscope is inserted through a tear in the intestine.

There is also a risk of perforation (a hole in the wall of the intestine) associated with colonoscopy. This risk is increased if the colonoscope is inserted through a tear in the intestine.

There is a small risk of reaction to the sedative used during colonoscopy. Reactions to the sedative may include:

- Drowsiness

- Nausea

- Vomiting

- Headache

If you experience any of these reactions, you should call your doctor.

In general, colonoscopy is a safe and effective medical procedure. Complications from colonoscopy are rare and usually minor.

What exactly happens during a colonoscopy?

During a colonoscopy, a doctor will insert a long, thin tube called a colonoscope into your rectum. The colonoscope has a tiny camera at the end of it, which allows the doctor to see the inside of your colon. They will then be able to look for any abnormal growths or polyps.

The colonoscope also has a tool on the end of it, which the doctor can use to remove any polyps that they find. Once the polyps have been removed, they will be sent off for further testing to see if they are cancerous.

The colonoscope can also be used to take biopsies of any abnormal areas that the doctor sees. A biopsy is a small sample of tissue that is taken from the body so that it can be tested for diseases.

The entire procedure usually takes around 30 minutes to an hour. You will be given a sedative before the procedure so that you will not be aware of what is happening. You may also be given a painkiller to help with any discomfort you may feel.

After the procedure, you will be monitored for a short period of time before being allowed to go home. It is important to drink plenty of fluids and eat a light diet for the rest of the day. You may experience some cramping and gas for a day or two after the procedure.

How will I feel day after colonoscopy?

Most people report that they feel much better the day after a colonoscopy than they did the day of the procedure. This is likely due to the fact that the procedure is over and they can finally relax. However, some people may still feel a bit groggy from the sedative they were given during the colonoscopy. It is important to not drive or operate heavy machinery until the effects of the sedative have worn off.

Some people may experience mild cramping or bloating after a colonoscopy. This is normal and should subside within a day or two. If you are feeling pain that is more severe, or if you are experiencing fever, chills, or rectal bleeding, you should contact your doctor.

It is also important to drink plenty of fluids and eat a high-fiber diet after a colonoscopy, as this will help ensure that your bowels are working properly.

Can I go to work day after colonoscopy?

A colonoscopy is a medical procedure where a doctor inserts a long, thin tube into the rectum and colon to check for any abnormalities or growths. It is generally considered safe and has a very low risk of complications. After the procedure, you may experience some cramping and bloating as your body adjusts to the tube. You will likely be able to go back to work the next day, but you may want to take it easy and rest as much as possible.

At what age is a colonoscopy recommended?

A colonoscopy is a diagnostic procedure that allows a doctor to evaluate the health of the large intestine (colon) and rectum. The colonoscopy can also be used to screen for cancer, as well as to detect and remove any abnormal growths in the colon.

The American Cancer Society recommends that people at average risk of colon cancer should begin colon cancer screening at age 45. African Americans, those with a family history of colon cancer, and people with certain other risk factors may need to start colon cancer screening at an earlier age.

During a colonoscopy, a flexible, lighted tube (colonoscope) is inserted into the rectum. The colonoscope is then passed through the entire length of the colon. The doctor is able to see the lining of the colon and look for any abnormal areas. If any are found, the doctor can then remove a small tissue sample (biopsy) for further testing.

In some cases, a colonoscopy may be used as a treatment. For example, if an abnormal growth is found, the doctor may remove it during the procedure. In other cases, the doctor may use the colonoscope to dilate (stretch) a narrowed section of the colon.

Most people tolerate colonoscopy well. However, the procedure may cause some cramping or bloating. Sedation is usually given during the procedure to help reduce any discomfort.

After a colonoscopy, it is important to drink plenty of fluids and eat a light diet for the rest of the day. People usually return to their normal diet and activities the following day.

What is the most common complication after colonoscopy?

The most common complication after colonoscopy is bleeding from the site where the biopsy was taken. Other complications can include:

- Infection

- Perforation (hole) in the colon

- Reaction to the sedative used during the procedure

Most of these complications are rare and can usually be treated successfully.

The colonoscopy is a widely used tool for colon cancer screening, but patients often have questions about the procedure. This article discusses some of the most common questions about colonoscopies, including what the procedure is, what to expect during and after the procedure, and what the risks are.

Will I stop pooping after a colonoscopy?

Patients frequently wonder if they will stop having bowel movements after a colonoscopy. The short answer is no, you will not stop having bowel movements after a colonoscopy.

During a colonoscopy, a long, flexible tube is inserted into the rectum and passed through the colon. A tiny camera at the end of the tube allows the doctor to view the inside of the colon. The colon is often gently inflated with air during the procedure to help the doctor get a clear view.

Some people experience bloating, gas, or cramping after a colonoscopy. This is often due to the air that is used to inflate the colon. These symptoms usually go away quickly.

It is important to remember that you will still have bowel movements after a colonoscopy. In fact, it is important to have a bowel movement after a colonoscopy so that any stool that was dislodged during the procedure can be passed.

You may be given a laxative to help you have a bowel movement after the procedure. You may also be advised to eat a high-fiber diet and drink plenty of fluids to help keep your bowel movements regular.

Do you have to take all your clothes off for a colonoscopy?

No, you do not have to remove all of your clothes for a colonoscopy. You will be asked to remove any clothing that will interfere with the procedure, such as belts or clothing with zippers. You will be given a gown to wear during the procedure.

What diseases can be detected by a colonoscopy?

A colonoscopy is a diagnostic procedure during which a doctor inserts a flexible tube with a camera attached into the rectum and large intestine. This allows the doctor to examine the inside of the intestine for any abnormalities, such as polyps or cancer.

Many different diseases can be detected during a colonoscopy. Some of the more common conditions that can be found during a colonoscopy include:

* colon cancer

* Crohn's disease

* ulcerative colitis

* polyps

Other less common conditions that might be found during a colonoscopy include:

* irritable bowel syndrome

* celiac disease

* diverticulitis

If any abnormalities are found during the colonoscopy, the doctor may recommend further testing or treatment. In some cases, a biopsy (tissue sample) may be taken during the colonoscopy.

What should you not do after a colonoscopy?

It is important to take it easy after a colonoscopy and give your body time to recover. There are a few things you should not do after the procedure.

You should not resume strenuous activity or exercise immediately after a colonoscopy. Take it easy for the rest of the day and resume your normal activity level the following day.

You should not drink alcohol or take non-prescription drugs for at least 24 hours after a colonoscopy. Alcohol can dehydrate you and non-prescription drugs may interact with the sedatives used during the procedure.

You should not drive for at least 24 hours after a colonoscopy. The sedatives used during the procedure can impair your ability to drive.

You should not make any major decisions for 24 hours after a colonoscopy. The sedatives used during the procedure can impair your ability to think clearly.

You should not drink anything with caffeine for 24 hours after a colonoscopy. Caffeine can dehydrate you.

Can polyps come out in your stool?

A colonoscopy is a diagnostic procedure in which a doctor inserts a long, flexible tube into the rectum and colon in order to examine the lining of these organs. This procedure allows the doctor to look for abnormalities such as lesions, polyps, or tumors.

Polyps are growths that occur on the lining of the colon or rectum. Some polyps are benign, meaning they are not cancerous. However, other polyps can develop into cancer over time. It is important to remove polyps during a colonoscopy in order to prevent them from becoming cancerous.

During a colonoscopy, the doctor may remove small polyps by snaring them with a wire loop and then cutting them away. Larger polyps may require surgery to remove. After the polyp is removed, it will be sent to a laboratory for testing.

It is possible for polyps to be passed out in the stool. However, it is more likely for benign polyps to be passed out in the stool than cancerous polyps. If you have had a colonoscopy and are concerned that a polyp may have been passed in your stool, you should contact your doctor.

Does your bottom hurt after a colonoscopy?

It is not uncommon to experience bloating and some abdominal pain after a colonoscopy. This is caused by the air that is used to inflate the colon during the procedure. The discomfort is usually mild and goes away within a day or two. If you are experiencing severe pain or bleeding, please contact your doctor.

What happens if they find cancerous polyps during a colonoscopy?

If cancerous polyps are found during a colonoscopy, the doctor will remove them. This is usually done by snipping them off with a special tool. The polyps are then sent to a lab to be checked for cancer. If the polyps are cancerous, the doctor will talk to the patient about treatment options.

Is it better to have a colonoscopy in the morning or afternoon?

There is no definitive answer to whether it is better to have a colonoscopy in the morning or afternoon. Some factors that could affect this decision include the patient's schedule and preference, the doctor's schedule, and the availability of the procedure.

Patients may prefer to have their colonoscopy in the morning so that they can get the procedure over with and not have to think about it for the rest of the day. Alternatively, some patients may prefer to have the procedure in the afternoon so that they have the rest of the day to recover. The doctor's schedule may also influence when the procedure is scheduled. If the patient is only available in the morning and the doctor has afternoon slots open, the procedure will likely be scheduled for the morning. Lastly, the availability of the procedure could also play a role. If there are more afternoon slots open for colonoscopies, the patient may be scheduled for that time.

There is no clear answer as to whether it is better to have a colonoscopy in the morning or afternoon. Ultimately, it is up to the patient and doctor to decide what time works best based on their schedules and preferences.

What are the signs of needing a colonoscopy?

There are a few signs that may indicate a need for a colonoscopy. If you experience any persistent changes in your bowel habits, such as diarrhea, constipation, or a change in the consistency of your stool, this could be a sign that something is wrong and you should speak to a doctor. Other signs include rectal bleeding, blood in the stool, and cramping or abdominal pain. If you have any of these symptoms, it is important to speak to a medical professional to determine if a colonoscopy is necessary.

Do females need colonoscopy?

As women, we are often told that we need to have regular Pap smears in order to check for cervical cancer. However, there is another cancer screening test that is just as important for women to have, and that is a colonoscopy.

So, do females need colonoscopy? The answer is yes, all women over the age of 50 should have a colonoscopy. This is because the risk of developing colon cancer increases with age. In fact, colon cancer is the third leading cause of cancer death in women.

There are a number of reasons why a colonoscopy is important for women. First, it can help to detect colon cancer at an early stage, when it is most treatable. Second, a colonoscopy can also help to identify precancerous polyps, which are growths that could eventually develop into cancer. Removing these polyps can help to prevent colon cancer from developing.

Finally, a colonoscopy is important because it is currently the only way to screen for colorectal cancer. This type of cancer can be difficult to detect, so it is important to have this screening test.

If you are over the age of 50, or if you have any risk factors for colon cancer, such as a family history of the disease, be sure to talk to your doctor about getting a colonoscopy. It could save your life.

Can I avoid a colonoscopy?

A colonoscopy is a procedure to evaluate the large intestine (colon) for inflammatory bowel disease, colorectal cancer, and other conditions. The colonoscope is a thin, flexible, lighted tube that is inserted into the rectum and passed through the colon. The colonoscope allows the doctor to see the lining of the colon and to remove tissue samples (biopsy) for testing if needed. Colonoscopy is considered the best test for diagnosing and evaluating many problems of the large intestine.

Most people with symptoms of colorectal cancer or inflammatory bowel disease will need a colonoscopy. The decision to have a colonoscopy is sometimes made without any symptoms, as a colonoscopy can also be used as a screening test for cancer or precancerous lesions in people without any symptoms. Screening is recommended for people starting at age 50 who are at average risk for colorectal cancer. People at high risk for colorectal cancer (for example, those with a family history of the disease) may need to start screening at a younger age.

There is no sure way to prevent colorectal cancer. However, there are some things you can do that may lower your risk, such as:

-Quit smoking

-Limit alcohol intake

-Exercise regularly

-Eat a diet high in fruits, vegetables, and whole grains

-Maintain a healthy weight

-Get vaccinated against the human papillomavirus (HPV)

-Get regular screenings for colorectal cancer

While there is no sure way to prevent colorectal cancer, you can lower your risk by making lifestyle changes and getting regular screenings.

What is the difference between colon cancer and colorectal cancer?

In short, colon cancer and colorectal cancer are two different types of cancer that can affect the large intestine (colon) and the rectum. While they may share some similarities, there are also some important differences between the two.

For starters, colon cancer typically affects the lower part of the colon, while colorectal cancer can affect the entire colon. Additionally, colon cancer is usually found in older adults, while colorectal cancer can affect people of any age.

Colon cancer and colorectal cancer also differ in their symptoms. Some common symptoms of colon cancer include blood in the stool, a change in bowel habits, and abdominal pain. On the other hand, common symptoms of colorectal cancer may include bleeding from the rectum, a change in stool size or shape, and cramping.

Finally, while there are a number of risk factors that can increase your chance of developing either type of cancer, there are some factors that are specific to colon cancer or colorectal cancer. For example, a family history of colon cancer or colorectal cancer is a risk factor for both, but eating a diet high in fat and red meat is a risk factor specifically for colon cancer.

While there are some key differences between colon cancer and colorectal cancer, it's important to remember that they are both serious diseases that can have a significant impact on your health. If you have any concerns about your risk of either type of cancer, be sure to talk to your doctor.

What do colon and rectal cancer have in common?

Cancer of the colon and rectum is often lumped together because they share many characteristics. However, there are some important distinctions between these two types of cancer.

For instance, colon cancer typically affects the older population, while rectal cancer is more common in younger people. In terms of risk factors, both colon and rectal cancer are linked to a diet high in red and processed meats, but colon cancer is also linked to a sedentary lifestyle and obesity, while rectal cancer is linked to smoking and heavy alcohol consumption.

There are also some differences in the symptoms of colon and rectal cancer. Colon cancer may cause bleeding from the rectum, a change in bowel habits, or abdominal pain, while rectal cancer may cause bleeding from the rectum, changes in bowel habits, or blood in the stool.

treatment options for colon and rectal cancer are similar, but there are some important differences. Surgery is the primary treatment for both types of cancer, but radiation therapy is typically only used for rectal cancer. Chemotherapy is often used for both types of cancer, but it is typically more effective for colon cancer.

In general, the prognosis for colon cancer is better than the prognosis for rectal cancer. The five-year survival rate for colon cancer is about 65%, while the five-year survival rate for rectal cancer is about 55%. However, the outlook for both types of cancer is improving, thanks to advances in treatment.

What are the signs and symptoms of colon cancer?

The most common sign of colon cancer is bleeding from the rectum or blood in the stool. However, bleeding may also be caused by other conditions, so it is important to see a doctor if you experience this symptom. Other potential signs and symptoms of colon cancer include:

- severe abdominal pain

- weight loss

- fatigue

- change in bowel habits

- anemia

If colon cancer is detected at an early stage, it is often treated successfully. However, if it is not detected early, it can spread to other parts of the body and be difficult to treat.

What is bowel cancer?

Bowel cancer, also known as colorectal cancer, is a cancer that starts in the large intestine (colon) or the rectum (end of the colon). Other types of cancer can start in the colon or rectum, but these are much less common. Cancer that starts in the colon may grow through the colon wall and spread to nearby lymph nodes. From there, it can travel to other parts of the body, such as the liver or lungs. Cancer that starts in the rectum is more likely to spread to the nearby lymph nodes. From there, it can travel to other parts of the body, such as the liver or lungs.

There are two main types of bowel cancer:

- Colon cancer: This is cancer that starts in the large intestine.

- Rectal cancer: This is cancer that starts in the rectum.

Bowel cancer is a common cancer, with more than 41,000 people diagnosed with it each year in the UK. It is the fourth most common cancer in men and the third most common cancer in women. The lifetime risk of developing bowel cancer is about 1 in 20 for men and 1 in 22 for women. This means that, on average, 1 in every 20 men and 1 in every 22 women in the UK will develop bowel cancer during their lifetime.

The cause of bowel cancer is unknown, but there are some risk factors that can increase your chance of developing the disease. These include:

- Age: The risk of developing bowel cancer increases with age. More than 90% of all cases are diagnosed in people aged 60 or over.

- Smoking: Smoking increases the risk of developing bowel cancer.

- Diet: A diet high in red or processed meats (such as bacon, ham and sausage), and low in fibre (found in wholegrain bread, fruits and vegetables), can increase your risk of bowel cancer.

- Obesity: Being obese or overweight can increase your risk of bowel cancer.

- Alcohol: Drinking alcohol can increase your risk of bowel cancer.

- Family history: If you have a family history of bowel cancer, you are more likely to develop the disease yourself.

- Previous history of cancer: If you have had cancer in the past, you are more likely to develop bowel cancer.

- Inflammatory bowel disease: Inflammatory bowel disease, such as Crohn's disease or ulcerative colitis, can increase your risk of bowel cancer.

If you have any of these risk factors, it does not mean that you will definitely develop bowel cancer. Many people with one or more of these risk factors never develop the disease.

What are the 10 early signs of colon cancer?

1. Abdominal pain, especially on the left side

2. Changes in bowel habits, such as diarrhoea, constipation or feeling that the bowel does not empty completely

3. Blood in the stool

4. Narrowing of the stool

5. Rectal bleeding

6. Fatigue

7. Weight loss

8. Unintended loss of muscle mass

9. Anemia

10. Family history of colon cancer

What are the early signs of bowel cancer?

Bowel cancer, also known as colorectal cancer, is a type of cancer that affects the large intestine (colon) and the rectum. The early signs of bowel cancer can be difficult to detect, as they may be similar to other common gastrointestinal disorders such as hemorrhoids, ulcerative colitis, and Crohn's disease.

One of the earliest signs of bowel cancer is bleeding from the rectum or blood in the stool. This bleeding may be severe or it may be so light that it goes unnoticed. Other early signs include a change in bowel habits, such as Diarrhea, constipation, or a feeling that the bowel does not empty completely.

Other early symptoms of bowel cancer may include:

- abdominal pain

- bloating

- gas

- nausea

- fatigue

- weight loss

If you experience any of these symptoms, it is important to see a doctor for a diagnosis. Early detection is crucial for the successful treatment of bowel cancer.

What are the two types of bowel cancer?

There are two types of bowel cancer: cancer of the colon and cancer of the rectum. Both types of cancer can be difficult to detect early, but colon cancer is usually easier to treat when it is caught early. Symptoms of bowel cancer can include bleeding from the rectum, a change in bowel habits, and pain in the abdomen. If you have any of these symptoms, it is important to see a doctor so that the cause can be found and treated.

Cancer of the colon is the most common type of bowel cancer. It occurs when cancer cells form in the lining of the colon. The colon is a long, tube-like organ in the digestive system that absorbs nutrients from food and eliminates waste. Cancer of the colon can grow slowly or quickly, and it can spread to other organs in the body, such as the liver.

Cancer of the rectum is the second most common type of bowel cancer. It occurs when cancer cells form in the lining of the rectum. The rectum is the last part of the large intestine. Cancer of the rectum can also grow slowly or quickly and spread to other organs in the body.

Treatment for bowel cancer depends on the stage of the cancer. Early stage cancer can often be treated with surgery. More advanced cancer may require radiation therapy, chemotherapy, or a combination of these treatments.

How long can you have colon cancer before noticing?

It is estimated that more than 95% of colorectal cancers develop from adenomatous polyps. These are growths on the inner wall of the colon or rectum that may become cancerous. The problem with adenomatous polyps is that they can take years, even decades, to develop into colon cancer. This is why colon cancer is often referred to as a "silent killer".

Most people with small adenomatous polyps will never develop colon cancer. However, those with a family history of the disease, or who have other risk factors, such as inflammatory bowel disease, are more likely to develop colon cancer from adenomatous polyps.

The good news is that, with regular screenings, colon cancer can be detected early, before it has a chance to spread. The best way to screen for colon cancer is with a colonoscopy. This is a procedure in which a doctor inserts a long, flexible tube with a camera into the rectum and colon. The doctor can then look for polyps or other signs of cancer.

If you are over the age of 50, or have a family history of colon cancer, it is important to talk to your doctor about getting a colonoscopy.

Where is colon cancer pain felt?

Colon cancer pain is typically felt in the lower abdomen, around the belly button. However, it can also be felt in the lower back, pelvis, and even in the rectum. The pain is often described as a dull ache or pressure, but it can also be sharp and cramp-like. It is important to note that not all colon cancers cause pain, so if you are experiencing pain in the abdomen, it is important to consult your doctor to rule out other possible causes.

What is the biggest symptom of colon cancer?

The biggest symptom of colon cancer is uncontrolled bleeding from the rectum or anus. This bleeding can be caused by a tumor in the colon or rectum that is eroding the blood vessels in the area. The bleeding can also be caused by a polyp that has become detached from the wall of the colon. Polyps are growths that can become cancerous over time.

Does colon cancer hurt when pressed?

There are a lot of questions that people have about colon cancer, and one of the most common is whether or not it hurts when pressed. The answer to this question can vary depending on the individual, but in general, the answer is no, colon cancer does not typically hurt when pressed. There are a few exceptions to this, however, such as if the cancer is in the rectum or anal area, as this can sometimes cause discomfort. Other than that, though, most people with colon cancer will not experience any pain when the area is pressed.

What does bowel cancer stools look like?

The most common symptom of bowel cancer is bleeding from the rectum or blood in the stool. However, bleeding may also be caused by other conditions, such as hemorrhoids. Therefore, it is important to see a doctor if you experience any rectal bleeding. Other symptoms of bowel cancer can include:

-A change in bowel habits, such as diarrhea, constipation, or a change in the consistency of the stool

-Abdominal pain

-Loss of appetite

-Unexplained weight loss

Blood in the stool or rectal bleeding can be a sign of bowel cancer. However, it is important to remember that other conditions, such as hemorrhoids, can also cause these symptoms. If you experience any rectal bleeding, it is important to see a doctor so that the cause can be determined. Other symptoms of bowel cancer can include changes in bowel habits, abdominal pain, loss of appetite, or unexplained weight loss. If you experience any of these symptoms, it is important to see a doctor so that the cause can be determined.

What is the main cause of colon polyps?

It is not fully understood what the main cause of colon polyps is. However, there are many theories and risk factors that are associated with the development of these growths.

One theory is that colon polyps are caused by a build-up of toxins in the colon. This build-up of toxins occurs when the colon is not able to efficiently remove waste from the body. The theory states that over time, these toxins begin to damage the cells of the colon, which leads to the formation of polyps.

Another theory is that colon polyps are caused by a chronic inflammation of the colon. This inflammation is thought to be caused by a number of different factors, including an unhealthy diet, a sedentary lifestyle, and stress. Chronic inflammation of the colon can damage the cells of the colon and lead to the development of polyps.

There are also a number of risk factors that are associated with the development of colon polyps. These risk factors include age, family history, smoking, and certain medical conditions.

AGE: The risk of developing colon polyps increases with age. This is thought to be due to the accumulation of toxins in the body over time.

FAMILY HISTORY: People who have a family history of colon polyps are more likely to develop them themselves. This suggests that there may be a genetic component to the development of colon polyps.

SMOKING: Smoking is a risk factor for the development of colon polyps. This is thought to be due to the harmful effects of smoke on the cells of the colon.

MEDICAL CONDITIONS: Certain medical conditions, such as Crohn's disease and ulcerative colitis, are associated with an increased risk of developing colon polyps. This is thought to be due to the chronic inflammation that is associated with these conditions.

While the exact cause of colon polyps is not known, there are many theories and risk factors that are associated with their development.

When should you worry about colon polyps?

Colon polyps are growths on the lining of the colon or rectum. Most colon polyps are benign, which means they are not cancerous. However, some types of colon polyps can develop into cancer. It is important to have colon polyps checked by a doctor so that any that may be cancerous can be removed before they turn into cancer.

Some colon polyps grow slowly and may never cause any problems. Others grow quickly and may turn into cancer. It is not always possible to know which type of colon polyp you have. This is why it is important to have colon polyps removed when they are found.

There are a few things that can increase your risk of developing colon polyps. These include:

- Family history. If you have a family member with colon polyps or colon cancer, you are more likely to develop colon polyps.

- Age. Colon polyps are more common in older adults.

- Diet. Eating a diet that is high in fat and low in fiber may increase your risk of developing colon polyps.

- Obesity. Being obese or overweight may increase your risk of developing colon polyps.

If you have any of these risk factors, it is important to talk to your doctor so that you can be screened for colon polyps. Screening for colon polyps can be done with a colonoscopy. This is a test that allows the doctor to look inside your colon and remove any polyps that are found.

If you have colon polyps, it is important to have them removed. This can help to prevent colon cancer.

Do colon polyps need to be removed?

A colonoscopy is a procedure in which a doctor inserts a long, flexible tube with a camera attached into the rectum and colon. This allows the doctor to examine the inside of the colon for any abnormal growths or polyps.

While many polyps are harmless and don't require treatment, some polyps can develop into cancer. For this reason, your doctor may recommend removing any polyps that are found during a colonoscopy.

There are a few different ways that polyps can be removed during a colonoscopy. The most common method is called snare polypectomy. This involves using a wire loop to cut off the polyp and then remove it through the scope. Other methods include lasers, hot water, or electricity.

Some polyps are too large to be removed through a scope and will require surgery. If your doctor finds a polyp that they believe is cancerous, they may also recommend a biopsy, which is a sample of tissue that is removed and examined for cancer cells.

In most cases, removal of polyps during a colonoscopy can be done safely and without any complications. However, as with any medical procedure, there are some risks involved. These include bleeding, infection, and perforation of the colon.

If you have a polyp or are considering having a colonoscopy, talk to your doctor about the risks and benefits of the procedure.

What food causes polyps in the colon?

There is no definitive answer to this question as everyone's colon and digestive system is different. However, there are some common triggers that have been linked to the formation of polyps in the colon. These include a diet high in red meat and fat, a lack of fibre, and excessive alcohol consumption.

Polyps are growths that develop on the lining of the colon (also known as the large intestine). They are usually benign (non-cancerous), but in some cases, they can develop into colorectal cancer. It is estimated that around 1 in 4 people in the United States will develop at least one polyp during their lifetime.

There are a number of factors that can increase your risk of developing colon polyps, including: age, family history, smoking, obesity, and certain inflammatory bowel diseases. While you may not be able to change some of these factors (e.g. age, family history), there are lifestyle changes you can make to help lower your risk.

Making dietary changes is one of the most effective ways to reduce your risk of colon polyps. As mentioned above, a diet high in red meat and fat can trigger the formation of polyps. Try to eat more lean protein, such as chicken or fish, and include plenty of fruits, vegetables, and whole grains in your diet. These foods are high in fibre, which has been shown to promote a healthy digestive system and may help reduce the risk of colon polyps.

In addition to dietary changes, maintaining a healthy weight is also important. Obesity is a risk factor for colon polyps, so aim to maintain a healthy body weight through exercise and a balanced diet. And finally, limiting your alcohol intake can also help reduce your risk of colon polyps. If you do drink alcohol, aim for no more than one drink per day for women and two drinks per day for men.

Finally, a diet that is low in fiber and high in processed foods is also thought to be a major contributing factor to the development of polyps. A diet that is low in fiber slows down the movement of food through the digestive system, which can lead to the buildup of toxins and an increase in the risk of developing polyps. In addition, processed foods are often high in refined sugar and unhealthy fats, both of which can contribute to the formation of polyps.

If you are concerned about the development of polyps in your colon, there are a few dietary changes that you can make to lower your risk. First, try to limit your intake of refined sugar and red meat. Instead, focus on eating more fresh fruits, vegetables, and whole grains. These foods are high in fiber and nutrients, and can help to keep your colon healthy. In addition, be sure to drink plenty of water and get regular exercise. These lifestyle changes can go a long way in maintaining colon health and preventing the development of polyps.

What are the stages of bowel cancer?

There are four main stages of bowel cancer. They are as follows:

1. Early cancer: The cancer is limited to the inner lining of the bowel.

2. Locally advanced cancer: The cancer has spread through the bowel wall to nearby tissues.

3. Metastatic cancer: The cancer has spread to distant organs, such as the liver or lungs.

4. Recurrent cancer: The cancer has come back after treatment.

What is the life expectancy of someone with bowel cancer?

The life expectancy of someone with bowel cancer varies depending on a number of factors, including the stage of the cancer, the person's age, and their overall health. In general, the prognosis for bowel cancer is good, with the majority of people surviving for five years or longer after diagnosis.

The stage of the cancer, as determined by how far it has spread, is the most important factor in determining life expectancy. If the cancer is caught early, before it has spread beyond the bowel, the chances of a cure are very good. However, if the cancer has spread to other organs, such as the liver or lungs, the prognosis is much poorer.

Age is another important factor in determining life expectancy. For example, a 70-year-old with bowel cancer is likely to have a shorter life expectancy than a 40-year-old with the same disease. This is because cancer is more common in older people, and the older a person is, the more likely they are to have other health problems that can complicate treatment.

Overall health is also a important factor. People who are in good general health tend to do better after a diagnosis of bowel cancer than those who are not. This is because they are better able to tolerate treatment and are more likely to respond well to it.

There are a number of treatments available for bowel cancer, and the type of treatment a person receives will also affect their life expectancy. Surgery is the most common treatment for early-stage bowel cancer, and it can be successful in curing the disease. However, if the cancer has spread, surgery may only be able to extend life by a few months. Chemotherapy and radiotherapy can also be used to treat bowel cancer, and they may be able to improve the prognosis for people with more advanced disease.

In general, the life expectancy of someone with bowel cancer is good, with the majority of people surviving for five years or longer after diagnosis. However, the stage of the cancer, the person's age, and their overall health are all important factors that can affect the prognosis.

Can I live a normal life with bowel cancer?

A cancer diagnosis is always scary, but if you have bowel cancer, you may be wondering what your life will be like going forward. The good news is that many people with bowel cancer go on to live long and healthy lives.

Of course, treatment for bowel cancer can be difficult, and it may cause some side effects that can be hard to deal with. But there are ways to manage these side effects, and many people find that treatment doesn't have a major impact on their day-to-day life.

It's important to remember that everyone is different, and your experience of living with bowel cancer will be unique to you. But it is possible to live a normal life with bowel cancer.

Is bowel cancer curable?

Yes, bowel cancer can be curable, but the chances of a cure depend on the stage of the cancer when it is diagnosed. The earlier the cancer is detected, the more likely it is to be cured. If the cancer has spread to nearby lymph nodes or to other parts of the body, the chances of a cure are lower.

There are a number of treatments available for bowel cancer, including surgery, radiotherapy, chemotherapy and targeted therapy. The type of treatment recommended will depend on the stage of the cancer, the location of the tumour, the patient's age and general health, and personal preferences.

Surgery is the most common treatment for bowel cancer. The surgeon removes the section of the bowel containing the cancer, along with a margin of healthy tissue around it. The two ends of the bowel are then sewn together. If the cancer is in the early stages and has not spread, surgery may be all that is needed.

Radiotherapy uses high-energy beams of radiation to kill cancer cells. It can be used before or after surgery, or on its own if surgery is not possible.

Chemotherapy uses drugs to kill cancer cells. It can be given before or after surgery, or on its own if surgery is not possible.

Targeted therapy is a newer type of treatment that uses drugs to target specific molecules involved in the growth and spread of cancer cells.

The decision about which treatment to have is often a difficult one. It is important to discuss all the options with a healthcare team that includes specialists in bowel cancer.

Should I be worried about having polyps?

Polyps are growths that can occur on the lining of the colon or rectum. Most polyps are benign (noncancerous), but some can be cancerous. Polyps are usually found during a colonoscopy.

The vast majority of polyps are benign (noncancerous). However, some polyps can develop into cancer. The risk of cancer depends on the type of polyp. For example, small, flat, pancreatic polyps are less likely to be cancerous than large, pedunculated (stalk-like) colonic polyps.

There are several different types of polyps, which can be classified by their appearance under a microscope. The most common type of polyp is an adenomatous polyp, which is a growth that arises from the glandular cells of the colon. Adenomatous polyps can be further divided into several subtypes, depending on their microscopic appearance.

The majority of adenomatous polyps are benign, but some can develop into cancer. The risk of cancer depends on the size, shape, and histologic features of the adenomatous polyp. For example, adenomatous polyps that are large, have an irregular shape, and contain abnormal cells are more likely to be cancerous than small, flat adenomatous polyps.

If you have been diagnosed with polyps, you may be wondering if you should be worried about cancer. The answer to this question depends on several factors, including the type of polyp, the number of polyps, and the features of the polyp.

If you have a single, small, flat adenomatous polyp, the risks of cancer are low. However, if you have multiple polyps, or a single large, pedunculated adenomatous polyp, the risks of cancer are higher. Your doctor will discuss the risks of cancer with you and recommend appropriate follow-up tests based on the type and number of polyps that you have.

What are the signs of polyps in your colon?

There are a few different signs that you may have polyps in your colon. First, you may notice bleeding from your rectum or blood in your stool. This can happen if the polyp rubs against your anal canal or rectum, or if it bleeds on its own.Secondly, you may experience changes in your bowel habits, such as diarrhea, constipation, or narrowing of your stool. This is because the polyp is blocking part of your colon and preventing stool from moving through as easily. Lastly, you may feel abdominal pain, bloating, or fullness because of the polyp. If you notice any of these signs, it's important to see a doctor so they can diagnose and treat the problem.

Do polyps affect bowel movements?

Polyps are growths on the lining of the colon or rectum. Some polyps grow slowly and cause no problems, but others can grow quickly and become cancerous. Cancerous polyps usually do not cause symptoms until they grow large enough to bleed or block the intestine.

Most polyps do not affect bowel movements. However, large polyps can cause changes in bowel habits, such as diarrhea, constipation, or a change in the size, shape, or color of stools. If you have any of these changes, you should see your doctor.

Can a doctor tell if polyp is cancerous during

colonoscopy?

A colonoscopy is a medical procedure that allows a doctor to look inside the large intestine (colon) and rectum to check for any abnormal growths, such as polyps. Polyps are small, fleshy growths that can develop on the lining of the colon or rectum. While most polyps are benign (noncancerous), some polyps can develop into cancer over time.

During a colonoscopy, the doctor will insert a long, flexible tube with a tiny camera attached into the rectum and slowly guide it through the colon. As the camera moves along the colon, the doctor will look for any polyps or abnormal growths. If any polyps are found, the doctor will remove them and send them to a lab for further testing.

The doctor will also biopsy (take a small tissue sample) any suspicious areas to be checked for cancer. In most cases, the doctor will be able to tell if a polyp is cancerous or benign based on its appearance. However, if the polyp is small or there is any concern that it might be cancerous, the tissue sample will be sent to a lab for further testing.

How normal is it to find polyps during a colonoscopy?

Polyps are growths that develop on the lining of the colon or rectum. While most polyps are benign, or non-cancerous, some can develop into cancer over time. According to the American Cancer Society, it is estimated that about 1 in 10 colon polyps will become cancerous.

Most people with colon polyps will never develop cancer. However, because colon cancer can be asymptomatic in its early stages, screening for colon cancer via colonoscopy is recommended for people over the age of 50, or earlier if you have a family history of the disease.

During a colonoscopy, a thin, flexible camera is inserted into the rectum and passed through the colon. This allows the doctor to visually inspect the lining of the colon for any abnormal growths. If polyps are found, they can be biopsied or removed during the procedure.

It is not uncommon to find benign polyps during a colonoscopy. In fact, according to the Mayo Clinic, as many as 1 in 4 people over the age of 50 have colon polyps. The vast majority of these polyps will never develop into cancer.

However, if you are diagnosed with colon polyps, it is important to follow up with your doctor to ensure that they are being monitored. If you have a family history of colon cancer, you may be at increased risk and may need to be screened more frequently.

While it is normal to find colon polyps during a colonoscopy, it is important to talk to your doctor if you have any concerns. If you are diagnosed with colon polyps, be sure to follow up with your doctor to ensure that they are being monitored.

How large are polyps?

Polyps are small, spiked growths that can form on the lining of the colon. They are usually benign, but some can develop into cancer. The size of a polyp can range from a few millimeters to several centimeters. Some polyps may be so small that they can only be seen with a microscope.

What is IBS

irritable bowel syndrome (IBS) is a disorder that affects the large intestine. Symptoms include cramping, abdominal pain, bloating, gas, and diarrhea. IBS can be a debilitating condition, making it difficult to carry out daily activities. There is no cure for IBS, but there are treatments that can help to ease symptoms.

What is the main trigger of IBS?

The main trigger of IBS is unknown, but there are several possible causes, such as anxiety, stress, food sensitivities, and hormonal changes. These triggers can lead to the symptoms of IBS, which include abdominal pain, bloating, diarrhea, and constipation.

How can I help myself with IBS?

If you're one of the millions of Americans suffering from irritable bowel syndrome (IBS), you know that it can be a real pain (literally). IBS is a chronic condition that causes abdominal pain and cramping, as well as diarrhea, constipation, gas, and bloating. While there is no cure for IBS, there are things you can do to help manage the symptoms and get some relief.

First, it's important to understand that IBS is a complex condition and there is not one single cause. It is believed to be caused by a combination of factors, including genetic predisposition, abnormal gut motility, alterations in the gut microbiome, and changes in the way the brain and nervous system interact with the digestive system. This means that there is not one simple solution that will work for everyone.

That being said, there are some general lifestyle and diet changes that can help to improve symptoms for many people. For example, eating a diet that is low in FODMAPs (fermentable oligosaccharides, disaccharides, monosaccharides, and polyols) has been shown to be helpful for some people. FODMAPs are found in many common foods, including wheat, dairy, beans, and certain fruits and vegetables. Eating a low-FODMAP diet can be tricky, so it's important to work with a registered dietitian who can help you figure out which foods to avoid.

In addition to dietary changes, there are some other lifestyle changes that can help. Getting regular exercise can help to relieve symptoms, as can managing stress. relaxation techniques such as yoga, meditation, anddeep breathing can also be helpful.

Of course, everyone is different and what works for one person may not work for another. If you're struggling to manage your IBS, it's important to talk to your doctor. They can help you figure out what might be causing your symptoms and develop a treatment plan that is right for you.

How do you detect if you have IBS?

If you're experiencing symptoms like abdominal pain, cramping, bloating, gas, diarrhea, or constipation, you might have irritable bowel syndrome (IBS). IBS is a disorder that affects the large intestine, or colon. There are several ways to detect if you have IBS.

Your doctor will likely start by asking you about your symptoms and medical history. They may also perform a physical exam. In some cases, your doctor may order tests, like a stool sample, to rule out other conditions.

There are also some at-home tests you can try. The Bristol Stool Chart is a tool that can help you identify your stool type. This can be helpful in tracking any changes in your bowel habits. Keeping a food diary is another way to track any patterns in your symptoms. You may want to note when you experience symptoms, what you ate that day, and any other factors that may have contributed to your discomfort.

If you're experiencing symptoms of IBS, talk to your doctor. They can help you find ways to manage your symptoms and feel your best.

What foods usually trigger IBS?

There isn't a definitive answer to this question as different people can have different triggers. However, there are some common triggers that tend to be troublesome for a lot of people with IBS.

One trigger is eating too quickly. When you eat too fast, you can end up swallowing a lot of air. This can lead to bloating and gas, which can be uncomfortable and even painful for people with IBS.

Another trigger is eating foods that are high in fat. Fatty foods can be difficult to digest and can also lead to bloating and gas.

Certain types of carbohydrates can also trigger IBS symptoms. These include fructose, lactose, and sorbitol. Fructose is found in many fruits, honey, and some vegetables. Lactose is found in milk and other dairy products. Sorbitol is a sugar alcohol that's often used as a sweetener in sugar-free products.

Eating large meals can also be a trigger for IBS. It's generally best to eat small, frequent meals throughout the day instead of large meals.

There are other potential triggers as well, such as stress, change in routine, and certain medications. If you're not sure what's triggering your IBS symptoms, it might be a good idea to keep a food diary. This can help you to identify patterns and figure out which foods are causing problems.

What does your poop look like with IBS?

Your poop can tell you a lot about your health. If you have IBS, your poop may look different than someone without IBS. It may be thinner, have less color, and more mucus. The consistency may also be different, ranging from hard and dry to watery.

Floating stool is also common in people with IBS. This is because gas can build up in the intestines and make the stool float. Stools that are particularly oily or greasy can also be a sign of IBS.

If you have IBS, your poop may also smell different. This is usually due to the bacteria in the intestine that breaks down food. The odor may be mild or strong, and it can be unpleasant.

If you're concerned about your poop, talk to your doctor. They can help you figure out if you have IBS and what you can do about it.

What should you avoid with IBS?

There is no one-size-fits-all answer to the question of what to avoid with IBS, as each person's experience with the condition is unique. However, there are some common dietary triggers that many people with IBS find helpful to avoid. These include:

-Foods high in fat: Fatty foods can trigger IBS symptoms in some people, so limiting your intake may help.

-Foods high in fiber: For some people with IBS, fiber can actually aggravate symptoms. If this is the case for you, you may want to avoid high-fiber foods or speak to your doctor about supplements that can help.

-Spicy foods: Spicy foods can trigger symptoms in some people with IBS, so it may be helpful to avoid them.

-Carbonated drinks: Carbonated beverages can cause bloating and gas, which can be trigger IBS symptoms.

-Alcohol: Alcohol can also trigger IBS symptoms, so it is best to avoid it or limit your intake if you have the condition.

If you have IBS, it is also important to stay hydrated and to avoid dehydration, which can trigger symptoms. Drinking plenty of fluids, especially water, throughout the day can help.

In addition to dietary triggers, there are some other things that can trigger IBS symptoms. These include:

-Stress: Stress can be a trigger for IBS symptoms, so it is important to find ways to manage stress if you have the condition.

-Certain medications: Some medications can trigger IBS symptoms, so it is important to speak to your doctor about any medications you are taking.

-Hormone changes: Hormonal changes, such as those that occur during menstruation, can trigger IBS symptoms in some people.

If you are avoiding trigger foods and other triggers but are still experiencing symptoms, it is important to speak to your doctor. There are many treatments available for IBS, and your doctor can help you find the one that is right for you.

What is IBD

Inflammatory bowel disease (IBD) is a condition that causes chronic inflammation of the digestive tract. The two most common types of IBD are ulcerative colitis and Crohn's disease. IBD can be a very debilitating condition, causing symptoms such as abdominal pain, fatigue, weight loss, and diarrhea. IBD can also lead to more serious complications, such as intestinal bleeding and intestinal cancer.

There is no one definitive cause of IBD, but it is thought to be due to a combination of genetic and environmental factors. IBD is more common in developed countries, and seems to be on the rise in recent years. This may be due to increased awareness and diagnosis, but it is also thought that changes in diet and the gut microbiome may play a role.

There is no cure for IBD, but there are treatments available to help control the symptoms. These include medication, surgery, and lifestyle changes. IBD is a lifelong condition, and managing it can be a challenge. However, with proper treatment, many people with IBD are able to lead normal, active lives.

What is the main trigger of IBD?

The main trigger of IBD is believed to be a combination of genetic and environmental factors. Studies have shown that IBD is more common in people with certain genes, and that the disease tends to run in families.

It's thought that environmental factors, such as infections, might also play a role in triggering IBD. Some research has suggested that a type of bacteria called mycobacteria may be involved. mycobacteria are found in soil and water, and people can come into contact with them through contact with contaminated food or water, or through breathing in contaminated air.

It's thought that mycobacteria may cause IBD by damaging the lining of the intestines, which triggers an immune response. The immune response leads to inflammation, which can lead to the symptoms of IBD.

How can I help myself with IBD?

There are a number of things that you can do to help manage your IBD. Remember, each person is different, so what works for one person may not work for another.

First, it's important to follow your treatment plan. This may include medication, surgery, or other therapies. If you don't take your medication as prescribed, or if you skip appointments, your IBD may flare up.

Second, pay attention to your body. If you notice any changes in your bowel movements or other symptoms, be sure to tell your doctor.

Third, eat a healthy diet. This means avoiding trigger foods that can make your IBD worse. Everyone's triggers are different, so you may need to experiment to figure out what works for you. There are also special diets that can help some people with IBD, such as the low FODMAP diet.

Fourth, manage your stress. Stress can make IBD symptoms worse, so it's important to find ways to relax. This may include yoga, meditation, or deep breathing exercises.

Fifth, get enough sleep. Sleep is important for overall health, and it can also help manage stress.

Finally, don't hesitate to ask for help. IBD can be a lot to handle, and it's okay to ask for help from friends, family, or your doctor.

How do you detect if you have IBD?

Inflammatory bowel disease (IBD) is a general term used to describe disorders that cause inflammation in the colon or small intestine. There are two main types of IBD: Crohn's disease and ulcerative colitis.

Crohn's disease can affect any part of the gastrointestinal tract from the mouth to the anus, but most often it affects the small intestine or the large intestine. Ulcerative colitis, on the other hand, only affects the large intestine.

There are a few different ways to detect if you have IBD. Your doctor may start by asking about your medical history and symptoms. They may also recommend a physical exam.

Blood tests may be ordered to look for signs of inflammation or anemia. A stool sample may also be collected to look for evidence of bleeding or infection.

Imaging tests may be used to get a better look at the gastrointestinal tract. X-rays, CT scans, MRIs, and endoscopies are all possible imaging tests that could be ordered.

IBD is a chronic condition, which means that it usually lasts for a long time and may flare up at different points throughout a person's life. There is no cure for IBD, but there are treatments that can help to manage the symptoms.

What foods usually trigger IBD?

There is no single answer to the question of which foods may trigger IBD flares, as the answer may differ from person to person. However, there are some general dietary guidelines that may help to minimize flares. For example, it is generally recommended that people with IBD avoid processed foods, sugary foods, and dairy products. Additionally, people with IBD should make sure to eat plenty of nutrient-rich foods, such as leafy green vegetables, fruits, and lean protein sources. Everyone's body is different, so it is important to experiment with different dietary approaches to see what works best for you.

What does your poop look like with IBD?

inflammatory bowel disease (IBD) is a condition that results in inflammation of the digestive tract. This can lead to a range of symptoms, including abdominal pain, diarrhea, weight loss, and fatigue. The severity of these symptoms can vary from person to person.

One of the most noticeable symptoms of IBD is changes in your stool. Since IBD affects the digestive tract, it can cause changes in the way your body breaks down and absorbs food. This can lead to changes in the frequency, consistency, and appearance of your stool.

Here are some of the most common changes in stool that can occur with IBD:

-Frequent diarrhea: This is often the most distressing symptom of IBD. Diarrhea can be watery and/or bloody. It can be accompanied by cramping, bloating, and abdominal pain.

-Constipation: IBD can also cause constipation. This may be due to inflammation in the large intestine, which can slow down the movement of stool through the digestive tract.

-Urgency: The need to have a bowel movement can be sudden and urgent. This can be disruptive to your daily life and can cause anxiety.

-Inconsistency: IBD can cause your stool to be diarrhea, constipation, or a mix of both. Your stool may also be watery, bloody, or mucus-like.

-Abdominal pain: Pain in the abdomen is a common symptom of IBD. The pain may be dull or cramp-like. It is often worse after eating or having a bowel movement.

-Weight loss: IBD can lead to weight loss due to the loss of appetite, diarrhea, and malabsorption of nutrients.

-Fatigue: Fatigue is a common symptom of IBD, especially when the disease is active. The fatigue may be due to the loss of appetite, diarrhea, and not getting enough sleep.

If you are experiencing any of these symptoms, it is important to see your doctor. They can perform a physical exam and order tests to confirm a diagnosis of IBD.

What should you avoid with IBD?

When you have inflammatory bowel disease (IBD), it's important to avoid things that may trigger your symptoms. Some people with IBD find that certain foods make their symptoms worse, so it's best to avoid these. Dairy products, fatty foods, and spicy foods are common triggers. You may also want to avoid caffeine, alcohol, and artificial sweeteners. Some people find that stress makes their IBD symptoms worse, so it's important to find ways to manage stress. Some people find that certain medications, such as NSAIDs, can trigger their IBD symptoms. If you're taking medication for your IBD, be sure to talk to your doctor about any potential side effects.

Have Questions / Comments?

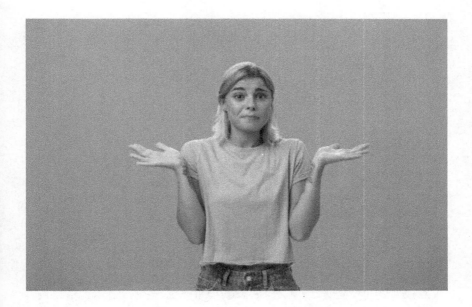

This book was designed to cover as much as possible but I know I have probably missed something, or some new amazing discovery that has just come out.

If you notice something missing or have a question that I failed to answer, please get in touch and let me know. If I can, I will email you an answer and also update the book so others can also benefit from it.

Thanks For Being Incredible :)

Submit Your Questions / Comments At:

https://BornIncredible.com/questions/

Get Another Book Free

We love writing and have produced a huge number of books.

For being one of our amazing readers, we would love to offer you another book we have created, 100% free.

To claim this limited time special offer, simply go to the site below and enter your name and email address.

You will then receive one of my great books, direct to your email account, 100% free!

https://BornIncredible.com/free-book-offer/

Also by Ethan D. Anderson

Printed in April 2023
by Rotomail Italia S.p.A., Vignate (MI) - Italy